Cracking
The Health and Happiness Code,
a Burn Out Antidote

*The 14 secrets on how to lower your stress, get
more energy, achieve more, be more productive
and have more fun in your life*

Adrian Ziliani

Cracking The Health and Happiness Code, a Burn Out Antidote

The 14 secrets on how to lower your stress, get more energy, achieve more, be more productive and have more fun in your life

By Adrian Ziliani

Published by: Herbalvalley GmbH, 9514 Wupepnau , Switzerland.
www.healthandhappinesscode.com

If you find any mistakes, send the error and page you found it on to my email AdrianZiliani@gmail.com

Dedication

This book is dedicated to all my friends, mentors, inspiring people and all coaches who helped me achieve happiness and excellence in my life.

It's also dedicated to my wonderful wife Mandy; who gave me two wonderful and healthy kids, Joshua and Matteo. Love you, Family!

Acknowledgements

To my parents, who gave me life and health, my humble childhood, my inspiration and drive to achieve more in life.

I am eternally grateful for my wife allowing me to follow my dreams and visions.

In my still young life, I had some experiences that made me the person I am today, and met people who inspired me. I know this was not by chance, but there is someone up in the sky, I call "my angel," that helped me be where I was supposed to be – at the right moment and the right time, and do the right thing at the right time. I am so grateful for all the positive energy that helped me achieve this major goal.

I made this quote by Anthony Robbins one of my life principles: No matter what happens in your life... "Life always happens for you and not to you!"

Disclaimer

This book is designed to provide general information on Health and Happiness only. This information is provided and sold with the knowledge that the publisher and author do not offer any legal or other professional advice. In the case of a need for any such expertise, consult with the appropriate professional. This book does not contain all information available on the subject. This book has not been created to be specific to any individual or organization's situation or needs. Every effort has been made to make this book as accurate as possible. However, there may be typographical and or content errors. Therefore, this book should serve only as a general guide and not as the ultimate source of subject information. This book contains information that might be dated and is intended only to educate and entertain. The author and publisher shall have no liability or responsibility to any person or entity regarding any loss or damage incurred, or alleged to have incurred, directly or indirectly, by the information contained in this book.

You hereby agree to be bound by this disclaimer or you may return this book within the guarantee time period for a full refund. If you find any mistakes, send the error and page you found it on to my email: AdrianZiliani@gmail.com

Thank you so much!

Foreword

As the Editor of Sacramento's Health & Fitness Magazine in California for over a decade, I have received and reviewed hundreds of books for our readers. Most of them are full of the latest and the greatest scientific theories on what to do to become healthier, based on medical knowledge, nutrition or fitness concepts, or psychological strategies.

What I liked most about Adrian's book is that he makes the process of becoming healthier and happier so simple. Why do we have to believe that anything and everything is complicated? Simplicity is always the best policy – and it works for staying happy. The more complicated we make things, the more stress we introduce into the equation.

Reading this book made me seriously analyze what was going on in my life from new angles that no one ever approached me about. For example, assessing one's social groups was a big one for me. I discovered that the source of my unhappiness was the people I spent the most time with. Adrian allowed me to realize that several people were in my life to take, take and take, and this situation will never lead to happiness. I had been thinking of them as a friend when in reality, they were not.

What a huge awakening it was for me, and just as soon as the awakening occurred, two new friends stepped into my life who were givers! Wow, I'm excited to be their friends! The book has made a huge impression on me and I am now thinking about my new friends in completely different ways. I think more about them as real people; not realizing that the damage done by the takers left a negative impression about people on me where I did not want to open the door to new friends.

When I first started reading the book, I kept thinking to myself, "Yes, that's true… nothing new here… yes, so what? I already know that." But this book was different than other books that had similar thoughts going through my head. There's some type of magic in this book that began rearranging the thoughts I had about the major areas of life contributing to happiness. I found myself actually thinking about the concepts without trying. A situation might arise and I viewed it through Adrian's eyes, not the same old ways I would usually view them.

This is truly an amazing ability for any author to have, and very few do. I urge you to consider this book as one that could truly transform your life. I can honestly say I'm happier after reading this book, and the seeds of happiness for the future have been successfully planted.

For many years I've been a retired chiropractor and still see nutrition clients. Many of them are unhappy for all sorts of reasons. I wish I had this book years ago to help them, as many of them could have transformed their life, too.

If you're debating whether or not to read this book, I will wholeheartedly encourage you to do it and embrace what's being stated in it. You have one thing to gain – your happiness – and it will be well worth it!

Adrian, excellent job and I can't wait to see life through your eyes with your next book, too! – Dr. Donna Schwontkowski, Retired Chiropractor, B.S. and M.S. Nutrition, Master's in Herbology, Editor of Health & Fitness Magazine, Sacramento, CA

Contents

Preface

Most importantly, I want to thank you for purchasing this book. I am very happy and honored to be your teacher and coach for the next days, weeks and months.

Why write or read a book about happiness and health? First of all, as a human, you deserve to be happy and have a healthy body. Secondly because… Well, it's a long story that started more than four decades ago in a beautiful little city in Switzerland.

Who I Am and How My Background May Be Like Yours in Some Ways

I was born in Lugano, a small city in the Italian part of Switzerland, a place where you have everything to be happy about and live a beautiful life. My parents were hard working. My father ran a restaurant and my mother worked in a Tea Room. They were always busy, arguing about money, and had to face the challenges of raising two kids and paying all the bills. As a result there was not so much happiness in our family.

When I was 3 years old, my parents got separated, and I grew up with my mother and brother. It was a painful time for me. I did not understand why this was happening to me and was mad at the world. My childhood was not very happy, and I was always asking myself why this happened to me and to my family. I was sad, unhappy, and back then I did not have the skill, mindset and tools of how to face this situation.

My Life Changed To Happiness with Ice Hockey

At the age of 15, I started to play ice hockey with a local team. I was so happy and proud of myself. I remember when I did my first training, I gave my all to show the trainer I was good enough, but I wasn't. My skating skills were weak compared to my teammates who were already skating for six or seven years. Luckily, there was still a position in the hockey team where you did not need to be a good skater, and there I was, the Goalkeeper!

I was so committed and proud to be part of a junior team that I trained harder than everyone else. I used ice hockey to increase my self-esteem, to experience joy and to find happiness. Ice hockey was my balance between high school and family, and it worked out well! I finally had a purpose in my life, and practicing a sport helped me forget where I came from. It became my source of happiness and joy.

Tony Robbins' Book Influences My Happiness Greatly

Finally, there was a way to be happy. Happiness and health were always my main driving forces in life, and at the age of 18, I purchased a book called "Unlimited Power" written by Tony Robbins. It was the Italian version, and that book was my salvation!

Every time a new challenge arose, I'd read it as my new bible. It worked all the way through high school and University. Today I am 45 years old, and when I think about the last 40 years of my life, I see many challenges, failures and achievements, but the only thing I was always driven to was happiness!

Our Busy Lives Don't Leave Room for Happiness

Happiness was missing in my parents' life and also in mine until I was 15. There is so much more need for happiness in our society – we are all so busy and stressed in our life we don't have time for it. Our career, family, and children absorb so much energy and time from our daily schedule. As a result, marriages fail, parents get burned out, and children grow up with weak role models, like I had to deal with.

This book is the result of my wisdom achieved in the last 30 years. It's fueled by the vision and hopes to inspire as many human beings as I can to become happier, more passionate and more balanced in their life. Today I describe myself as a successful and happy father and husband and businessman. So let's begin with the journey.

Introduction

Happiness is a state of mind that affects everything you do. You can be happier at home, in love, in your career, and in every other aspect of your life as long as you know what needs to be done to achieve happiness.

Have You Already Given Up on Happiness?

Many people give up on achieving happiness far too easily. They think that happiness is simply "not in the cards" for them.

If you have ever said this to yourself, you are denying yourself one of the simple pleasures in life that can be obtained. What will make you happy? First, it is all about creating realistic goals based upon where you are currently.

You may not be able to become the President of the United States – and will this really bring you happiness anyway? These are things that you need to realize if you want to become truly happy – and maintain it throughout your entire life.

Who doesn't want to be healthier and happier? You may be surprised by how easy it is to achieve and how once you have the skill, you can apply it to the rest of your life.

What You'll Discover in This Book

Let's list out all the things that they will gain from the book here. We start out with foods info but the first chapters are more about changing the mindset…

Throughout this book, you will discover the keys to being healthier through the foods you eat and even the various poisons you should avoid. Once you learn what's preventing you from being happy, the only direction you have to go is up!

There are many aspects that can have a dramatic effect on your life. You will learn about all of them, including focus, language, and physiology in the next chapters. By the time you reach the end of the book, you will know what you need to do to be happier and healthier – and to maintain it for a lifetime.

Forget about what you think you know about your health. You may be feeding poison into your body on a daily basis without even realizing it. This can leave you feeling less than good about yourself – and this isn't a feeling that you want to have. When you change the way you eat, you can change the way you feel, and think.

Within a short period of time, you may find that you have more energy, which brings about a better outlook about each day. More energy and a better outlook lead you to being more involved with family and friends and more grateful to be alive. With greater family involvement, your world is a great place to be – and your personality and overall sunny outlook on life will rub off on those around you, which is always a good thing. This will encourage more people to be close to you so you can be surrounded with those who have a similar outlook on life.

What is Happiness Really?

Happiness is not just about the food you eat. It's about what you focus on and the way you speak to yourself and others. Your mood is a powerful tool and when you are in a better mood, it will result in you being happier on a day-to-day basis.

You'll have to learn about your emotions, identify them, and know how to improve them so they never affect your ability to be happy. The sooner you learn to identify a problem emotion, the faster you can start to work on improving it.

Have you ever seen people walking down the street, smiling and just happy to be alive? Don't you wish that you had that happy attitude, too?

Happy people aren't taking any drugs to get this way and they haven't found some miracle serum to inject themselves with. They have simply learned the secrets behind being healthy and happy – and those same secrets are revealed through this book.

In this book, you'll have exercises to do that will begin to access your hidden happiness. Let's start with the first one now.

Exercise 1. Why Be Happy?

1. On a sheet of paper, write down 10 reasons why you want and deserve to be happy. Write each reason in bold capital letters.

2. Print it out. Look at it and read it aloud every day at least once. When you read it, say it out loud to engage your physiology. This process will help you keep the focus on why you want to be happy, and your brain will start recognizing what you want.

Chapter 1
Achieve the Proper Focus

"It is in your moments of decision that your destiny is shaped."
— *Anthony Robbins*

Examine Your Current Views of Happiness

What is your definition of happiness? Are you happy when you are with the person you love most in the world? Are you happy when you have a certain amount of money in your bank account? Are you happy when you get your way? Or are you happy when you spend time with your family?

Identify what makes you happy. You also have to be realistic about whether these things are actually making you happy or are simply make you feel a sense of satisfaction. There's a big difference between happiness and satisfaction. The sooner you identify the differences, the easier it will be to reach for happiness.

In order for all of this to happen, you need to have the proper focus. Focus on what is important to you and how you can be happy.

Happiness Equates to Peace Within Yourself

When you have a smile on your face, it is likely because you have the feeling of happiness coursing through your body. This can be because of five different things: 1) you are at peace with yourself, 2) you have reached a particular goal, 3) someone has said something pleasing to you, 4) you have taken actions to release endorphins in your body, or 5) because of something else.

Do Other People's Accomplishments Anger You?

The proper focus is a big key to the ability to achieve happiness. Many people are unhappy because they look around and name all the things they don't have. Whatever happened to being grateful for the things that you do have? **The focus should be on what you have already achieved and what you already have.** The moment you start looking elsewhere is the moment you lose that happy feeling.

Be grateful for what is going right in your life. This can include such things as your body, your family, your health, your career, and much more. When you have run out of things to be grateful for, just be grateful to be alive. Remember that it could always be worse, yet it's not because you are in the land of the living – and that is something to focus on and be thankful for!

Why Comparing Yourself to Others Is a Dead End

If you look to compare yourself with others, you will always be unhappy. You are a unique individual and therefore you cannot compare yourself to others. There is always going to be someone who is more attractive, makes more money or is more successful than you are, no matter who you are. Money isn't going to change that and neither is anything else.

You can only control your outlook on life so the comparisons have to stop. Making comparisons is one of the unhealthiest things you can do. You are not like anyone else. Just because someone has more money or is more attractive or is more successful does not mean that you are unable to reach happiness.

Define your happiness so it does not include a comparison to other people. This may seem difficult but not if you focus on the "you" of the equation. As soon as you introduce someone else into your definition of happiness, you have missed the entire point. You cannot achieve happiness if you are making comparisons.

Comparing Yourself to Others is Not Apples to Apples

When you compare yourself to someone else, you aren't comparing apples to apples. You can compare yourself to yourself, but that's it. You don't know the other person's background and what they had to do to get where they are today.

You don't know how they were able to go to the Ivy League school or how they "fell" into the position that they are in. You simply don't know the whole story and that makes it impossible for you to compare yourself to them. The only thing you can do is worry about you and what is going on in your life.

The Answer is Looking Inward, Not Outward

Since you cannot compare yourself to others, you can only look inward for your focus. Are you better or worse off than you were five years ago? What was going on five years ago that made your life better or worse? These comparisons are healthy because it is about you and where you have been and where you are going. These are the only comparisons that can and should be done because you are now comparing apples to apples.

You Will Gain the Tools to Change How You Think About Comparisons

I remember a time in high school when I used to compare my family and life to the ones of my school peers. We were so different. My friends at school had parents, money, and a family, and my situation was the opposite. I felt frustrated, mad at the world and at my parents. I was felt miserable. I was not comparing apples to apples.

Back then I was living at my mother's apartment, and as a 16-year-old boy, I did not have the tools and mindset to better understand this situation. Today I absolutely know that feeling happy and joyful can be achieved in a moment by focusing on everything I have in my life, including my health, my intelligence, my drive, my determination, my power to believe, my faith, and by just being alive!

Who Are You? Knowing Yourself Brings Happiness

You can become a better person with a little inner reflection. The more you know who "you" are, the easier it will be to make changes so you can achieve the happiness you have been chasing for so long.

Take a long look at who you are, what you have accomplished, and where you are headed. If you are unhappy in any of these aspects, begin creating goals to make improvements in these areas.

Are you unhappy with what you have accomplished? This is something that you need to think about. If you have not accomplished as much as you thought you would, think about what you would like to accomplish.

Would you like to go to college? Would you like to start a family? Any of these are possible and you can begin taking actions to accomplish these goals. Throughout this book, there will be guides to help you create effective goals and take action so you have the motivation necessary to drive you all the way through to the end result, even when there are obstacles in your way.

Gauge Your Life's Progress Right Now

If you are happier than you were five years ago, you know you are headed in the right direction. This should give you a sense of accomplishment and a little pep in your step. If you aren't happier than you were five years ago, take a step back and ask yourself why.

What has changed between then and now? What can you do to get back to that point? You have been there once, so once you learn what it is that has changed, you can make the change once again and return to the point of happiness.

Let's Make a Dream Chart/Progress Chart

You can always use a dream chart or a progress chart to see where you are and how far you have come. This can allow you to see what you have accomplished and will give you the "push" you need sometimes to take things a step further. You can only compare yourself to you and when you lose sight of what you have done and where you are heading, a chart on your wall can help to bring you back into line.

I did this exercise first when I was 21 and wrote down all my current achievements and the challenges I had to overcome. It was such a powerful moment and I remember I felt so strong and happy in a heartbeat. Since then, I revise that list on a regular base and just read it, or when I meditate, I visualize all I achieved in my life, and that's when magic happens!

Progress Chart Example

What are your achievements for your list? To give you an example, my Progress Chart listing a few achievements in my life is below. Thinking about them helps me stay strong and happy:

1989 Graduated from high school

1989 My first Ice hockey game with the professional team in my home-town, Lugano

1997 Graduated from the SFIT Swiss Federal Institute of Technology

1999 Ran my first NYC Marathon

2005 Founded my own company and bought my house

2006 Got married with my wonderful wife Mandy

2008 My first son Joshua was born

2012 My second son Matteo was born

2013 Wrote my first book

2015 Celebrate my 10th anniversary for my Company and published my second book

Focus Boards Keep Your Mind on Track

It may be helpful to create a "focus board" in your home or office. Place it somewhere where you can see it multiple times throughout the day. Put a few words up there for you to focus on with your subconscious mind during the day. Maybe you could focus on a particular upcoming event or focus on the fact that you just accomplished something really big.

What are you most proud of? There has to be something. Maybe you helped a friend meet the love of his or her life. Maybe you gave birth to an amazing child. Maybe you just got a scholarship to college.

Hold onto that thing that you are most proud of because no one can ever take it away from you. When you can hold onto your accomplishments, you will find that it is harder to compare yourself to others because no one has been able to accomplish the EXACT same thing as you. Your situation is always going to be unique.

Why You Are So Unique

Even if someone else won the same scholarship you did, you had a different background in order to achieve it. There were likely smaller milestones where you had to overcome things in order to win it.

Someone else who won the scholarship is not you. They did not go through the same things, physically, mentally, or emotionally. Don't downplay your accomplishments just because there are other people involved.

This is your chance to be a little selfish. It doesn't matter if 10 or even a hundred other people accomplished the same thing. YOU were the one that accomplished it and it's something to be proud of. As far as being better than someone (or someone being better than you), it goes back to not making comparisons to other people.

Eliminate other people from the equation. Whether you accomplish something that others have or not, it is still an accomplishment. Do not take that away from yourself. It doesn't matter if other people did it better or worse than you because you accomplished the goal.

You Become What You Focus On

Focus on what you can control and this is going to be a lot easier for you to manage. Why bother focusing on the things you cannot control? This type of thinking leads to frustration, aggravation, and stress. Those are three things in your life that will never make you happy, so it's easier to just avoid them so you can be happy.

Think about all the happy people in your life. They let things roll past them because they cannot change them. While it may be frustrating at first, learn to let certain things go. No matter how much you dislike them or want them to change, you are incapable of changing them. The sooner you realize these things, the easier it will be to get in the kind of mood that you want to be in – a happy one!

Learn What You Can Control and What You Can't

It's important to learn what you can and more importantly, what you cannot control. If you cannot identify what you can control, a significant amount of stress floods into your life. Then you'll spend precious energy trying to change things that cannot be changed. Your stress level rises dramatically and without realizing it, obstacles arise that are difficult to overcome.

Remember: You can control your focus. You can decide every day what to focus on – either what is not working and what you don't have and feel miserable, or on what to be grateful for in your life. If you choose the latter, your reward is feeling happy and balanced.

Do You Realize You are Already Rich?

You were born rich. You have two arms, two legs, a beautiful body perfectly working in balance. Your heart and organs are all connected and work all day long. Your brain is a supercomputer working for you on whatever you set your mind on. It's easy to feel grateful and happy!

I remember when my first son Joshua was born, it was 2:00 a.m., and the event was the most exciting, touching and emotionally moving experience of my life. Think about it: 9-1/2 months later after making love, a miracle happens! A baby is born, looking perfect, with all the organs working together.

After that experience, I realized life is a miracle and the greatest gift you can ever receive. So I often thank God for having the privilege to be alive, to walk, to see, to feel to touch and to talk. Being grateful is the fastest and easiest way to feel joy, happiness and love.

Before we get to the very end of this chapter, let's do to an exercise.

Exercise 2. You are Grateful!

1. What are you grateful for? Stop reading and write down at least 10 reasons you can be grateful for today.

2. Read this list every day for 1 week.

3. The next week, repeat the process, brainstorming and writing 10 additional reasons you are grateful. You'll be amazed at how suddenly, you begin to see all sorts of things to be grateful for!

By doing this consistently, you condition your mind to feel balanced, happy and relaxed.

Dealing With Difficult People is Easy With This New Philosophy

You cannot change other people or other situations. However, what you can control is how you deal with those people, how you interact with those people and how you deal with the situations. You can even change your mind about how you feel about the people.

Even the worst of situations can be dealt with in an upbeat way as soon as you realize that you are not the person to change the situation.

The Milk is Spilt – What Do You Do?

The old saying of not crying over spilled milk has a place in your life. The milk is already spilt. Crying over it is not going to suddenly go back in time and prevent the milk from being spilt. Crying about it will not improve the situation. On the other hand, you can clean up the milk and move past the spillage so that you can get more things done. The latter is the more productive response and the response to adopt for all obstacles in your life.

When you start to cry about something or feel frustrated about something, you are letting negativity in your life and you lose your focus. Your focus towards a particular goal is lost because your focus is on the obstacle. You are allowing the obstacle to win because you are spending more time on it than it deserves.

Commit To Your Original Focus No Matter What

The original focus needs to be maintained no matter what. Runners don't get bent out of shape when there is a rock on the track because they can't afford to.

It's an inconvenience and it may have even tripped them up but their focus is on reaching the finish line. If they stopped and concentrated on the rock, other runners would pass them by. They might not even reach the finish line because the obstacle has turned into their focus.

What To Do If You Don't Get That Much Desired Promotion

The proper focus needs to be centered on you and positive things. When something isn't positive, focus on making it into something positive. Teach yourself how to put a positive spin on things so you don't let your emotions get out of control.

You didn't get the promotion at work you really wanted. The good news is you don't have to work all those extra hours and you take on added responsibilities. You already know your current job position and you are good at it, so be a shining star within the company.

Being upset about not getting the promotion will not suddenly get you the promotion. If your boss sees you upset, do you think he will change his mind? Only worry about the things you can actually change so you can put a positive spin on negative events and move on.

Big Tip: Smile and It Changes Your Physiology!

Sometimes putting a smile on your face in the situations where you really want to cry can help. The smile is just as much physiological as it is physical. Smiling doesn't take a lot of effort and it can make you feel good as soon as you get those muscles working on your face.

Here's the good news: it takes less effort to smile than it does to frown. Due to the muscles involved with each facial expression, it's scientifically proven that it's easier to smile than to frown. Think about that the next time you want to frown because a situation has you feeling low. As soon as you smile, it may actually put you in a better mood, even if you have to force it out initially.

How to Use Priorities in Life to Achieve Mental and Emotional Balance

When you learn to focus on the positive things, you can do more, be more, and influence more. What's important in your life?

Achieve balance without one thing being considerably more important than another. If you put your job as the #1 priority, your family is going to take a back burner and that's not fair to you or them. To achieve balance, identify where your focus should be.

Happiness Occurs Naturally – How To Let It Happen

You don't have to work at being happy. It should happen naturally. This may seem impossible right now based upon what is going on in your life. You can smile and happiness can be yours. It doesn't matter who has more possessions than you or who has accomplished more than you. What matters is you and your circle of loved ones.

Create a Focus Board on Paper and In Your Mind

Your focus board, either physically or mentally, needs to be filled with positive emotions and positive actions. Put the focus on you and the things you can change instead of the people around you. Comparisons only work when they are apples to apples and you are an individual, so the comparisons can never work in your favor if they're about other people.

Remember that you are the only one who can control what you do. While other people may influence you, you are the one who determines whether you are going to listen to them or not. If you have someone who is constantly driving you down and trying to manipulate you, consider removing him or her from your life. If this person is your boss, it may help to sit down with him and discuss your point of view. If that does not work, consider getting a new job. Regardless of what goes on around you, there are ways for you to take control.

When Will You Realize How To Identify What's Important?

As soon as you learn that you can do more, be more, and influence more in your life, it will be easier to identify what is important. No one should or can answer these questions for you.

While your workplace may feel they are the most important, you are the one who ultimately makes this decision. For example, if you are trying to make your family the #1 priority, and your workplace is fighting vying for the #1 spot, the result is a considerable amount of unhappiness.

Two things are fighting at becoming the most dominant part of your life. If you give into your workplace, your family is not going to be happy. If you give into your family, your workplace may create a nightmare environment.

Need a bit more explanation about this here. Example: explain As a result of influential characters

As a result of influential characters, you may have to create new actions in order to set on the path of reaching happiness.

It may not be something that happens overnight. You may have to identify various paths that you can take in order to create a happy balance. There are plenty of workplaces that want you to establish a work/family balance. If your current workplace is not allowing you to establish this, you may want to start on a path that allows you to discover a new place of employment.

Additionally, communication will help you to establish what is and what is not working for you. If your family does not understand your need to go to work, you may have to explain it to them. By creating an open line of communication between all areas of your life, it will be easier for everyone to be on the same page. Once everyone is on the same page, they can support your need in achieving happiness without working so hard at it.

You control being happy and that means you control your overall health and well being. You can focus on being a happier, healthier person as long as you have the right mindset and the right tools.

Chapter 2
It's All About Language

"The words we attach to our experience become our experience."

— Anthony Robbins

Your Words Harm or Help You

The language you use on a regular basis will influence your happiness because it affects your mood. Regardless of whether you are talking to yourself or someone else, you want to be careful about the words used plus the way you say them. When you control the way you speak, you control your emotions and offer a better state of mind on an ongoing basis.

It doesn't matter if you are talking to yourself or others. What you say, regardless of to whom, shows how you are feeling and can give you a peek into the emotions felt at the moment. You may love someone to pieces but talk to them in a short, stressed mode. This means you are likely not at your happiest point. The person you are speaking to doesn't deserve this and what you say and how you say it is going to affect their mood, too.

Be cautious about how you speak because it matters. If you talk to yourself in a negative way, you are going to believe it. The same is true if you speak to others in a demeaning way on a regular basis. They may develop a low sense of self-worth simply because you are having a bad day. It's not fair to them. Be conscious about how powerful your words really are so you can censor yourself periodically.

Speaking to Yourself

Start analyzing the way you talk to yourself. Everyone talks to himself or herself during the day. When you look in the mirror, what do you think? What do you say out loud about yourself? When you meet someone and see what they have or find out what they are doing, your mind is busy making comments to yourself. As you prepare for a presentation at work or to meet someone for the first time, you mentally pump yourself up with a particular type of mojo.

It is important to speak to yourself in a positive way. How else would you talk to yourself? Many people think they only speak in a positive way but positivity may not be what's actually coming through because you are down on your luck, emotional, or holding onto some resentment for a particular person or event in your life.

Positive affirmations are a great way to pump you up and get yourself in a positive state of mind. You can repeat them out loud or to yourself throughout the day. Affirmations can be like mini mantras recited repeatedly. They help influence your emotions so you begin to believe the words that you are speaking.

Some examples of positive affirmations include:

I am worthy.

I can do anything I put my mind to.

I look really good today.

I am healthy and happy.

I am thankful for all that is going on in my life.

I am a smart and intelligent person and people value my opinion.

It is important to begin the phrase with "I am…" Then say exactly who you are, or who you want to become. By repeating your mantra or incantation every day, your unconscious mind will start to believe it, and as result, you behave as the person you want to become. You become that person.

Depending upon what you are trying to psyche yourself up to do, the affirmation can be anything you want it to be. It all goes back to being positive and learning to speak to yourself in a positive and healthy manner.

A Primer on Affirmations

There are countless websites with lists of affirmations. You can "borrow" these at any time so you have dozens of great examples of what to say when speaking to yourself.

Often the affirmations are reflective of the goals you want to achieve. One example of an affirmation to start with is an affirmation about self-worth. If you have low self-worth, use a mantra that states you have high self-worth. Do this even if you may not believe you need it right now.

If you want to lose weight, provide yourself with motivational mantras that provide you with motivation to continue. Some of them will be longer than others. You can write them down, record them, and even have friends and family members recite them to you. Use any mantra that works on a regular basis – these words of encouragement and positive action will then play through your head on a regular basis.

Start Your Day with A Positive Affirmation

A great way to start your day is to compliment yourself while in front of the mirror. Initially, this may seem vain but it's a way of improving your outlook and developing self-confidence. Choose something you like about yourself – your hair, skin, outfit; anything whatsoever. This will build yourself up so you feel more confident to tackle anything happening during your day. You will feel better equipped to handle any obstacles in your way so your focus doesn't disappear as soon as you are met with any kind of resistance.

When you learn how to speak to yourself in a positive manner, you can be sure you are making an impact on your overall emotions. You build yourself up instead of tearing yourself down and this is one of the most important things to do to achieve happiness.

Start first thing in the morning when you look at your reflection in the mirror. Tell yourself, "I'm a good-looking person" or "I look good!" and then continue by admiring a few of your features. This behavior gives you a boost of self-confidence and will affect how you carry yourself for the day. If you look in the mirror and criticize everything about yourself, your self-worth plummets. This will lead to feelings of inadequacy for the rest of the day and make it hard to smile, let alone be happy.

Filter Your Self-Talk – Are You Lying to Yourself?

You may not think you have to filter what you say to yourself, but you do. If you cannot talk to yourself in a positive manner, how will you say positive and upbeat things to anyone else? Change always starts within you. You are happier when you love yourself first. People around you will be happier when you are happy.

Self-worth and self-confidence are two of the most important feelings and if you don't have these in high levels, everything you do is affected – and not in a positive way. Low self-worth causes your goals to lag behind and makes you unhappy. Why? It's because you have convinced yourself you are not allowed to be happy or that happiness is not achievable.

In essence, you have lied to yourself. How did you do this? You talked to yourself in a negative way and put yourself down so much that every ounce of your being has bought into the lie.

Now is the time to start talking to yourself in a more positive way. You can be anyone you want to be. You are capable of changing yourself for the better. If you want to be a better person, all you have to do is make the decision to be. Later on in the next chapters, you will learn about the law of attraction and how this law can be used to help you.

Do You Believe Only Certain People Should Be Happy?

You can be a better, happier person. It's not true that the universe has deemed only certain people worthy of happiness and success. You can be just as happy as anyone else; you simply need to learn to talk to yourself in a more positive way. Pump yourself up motivationally and don't allow yourself to speak to yourself in a harsh way. Stop before you think about something in a negative way.

Start Thinking of Yourself as Great

What you hear from yourself has a stronger impact than anything else. You are a great person and you need to recognize this through and through. Don't compare yourself to others. To start thinking of yourself as great, look in the mirror and find one great thing about yourself. Focus on this on thing.

You are unique and your uniqueness creates the beauty in your body. Comparing yourself to others is the fastest way to make you unhappy and miserable.

Affirmations are Mantras and Incantations

I created an incantation I repeat on a daily basis. I condition my mind so I feel strong, happy, intelligent and wealthy. You can create an incantation or mantra by considering your values and beliefs. Do it. It will take about 30 minutes. Then use your incantation to pump yourself up.

These are my incantations I created by brainstorming my values and the person I wanted to become:

I am strong, driven and intelligent.

I am an amazing and successful businessman.

I am a passionate and loving husband and father.

I am wildly, wildly wealthy.

I am a Millionaire and have a Billionaire mindset.

Use Your Focus Board to Fuel Your Affirmations

Running out of great conversation to have with yourself? Go to your focus board of things that you have accomplished or want to accomplish. Borrow a few things to have the spirit to propel yourself forward and be a better, happier, healthier person. Reading various motivational books can also be very advantageous.

Various books on this topic have hit the New York Times bestseller list several times because of the message they deliver. You can read these over and over again, highlight important chapters, and teach yourself how to talk to yourself in a positive way. Positive thinking and positive speech helps you create a brighter outlook on life, allowing you to reach that level of happiness that you desire most in the world.

No Ego Here

It's not being egotistical to think that it's all about you because in this case, it IS all about you. It's important to get yourself in order before you can work on anything else. If you cannot talk to yourself in a positive manner, there is no way you will talk to anyone else positively – and this is absolutely critical.

It's important to accept and own yourself. Before you can love anyone else, you have to love yourself. To love yourself, start by owning your personality, habits, appearance, and everything else about you. Be comfortable in your own skin, as this will serve you well in life. It can be advantageous to develop a "love me or hate me" attitude.

If people don't love you, then you don't want them around. It's not healthy. Choose the people you want to be around; those who don't love you shouldn't be in the picture. The choice always comes back to accepting yourself. Deep down, identify every flaw – the physical, mental, and emotional ones, and tell yourself you are okay with them and love them. All these things are a part of you and you must love them all.

Are You Comfortable With Being Different?

It's okay to be different. Look at hipsters. As an individual, they may look a little unusual because they have chosen to wear something or do something out of the ordinary. This isn't because they're an unusual person. It's because they are comfortable enough with themselves to be who they are.

Sometimes they go for the ironic as a statement. They are being who they want to be, regardless of what other people think.

A sign of a healthy self-esteem is a person who does what he or she wants, wears what he or she wants to wear, and says what he or she wants to say. Stop caring so much about what others have to say and instead focus on you and loving yourself. Don't be a pleaser and don't be the person other people want to see, just to get acceptance. Be yourself, be authentic and be genuine.

Accept Yourself and Feel Happier

The moment you start accepting yourself – that is, all of yourself – it will be easier to achieve happiness. If you continue to find flaws, it's only a matter of time before happiness turns to sadness, anger or depression. Happiness will be a permanent part of your life once you accept and embrace every part of you. Your self-esteem will be at a healthy level and you can see improvements throughout all aspects of your life.

Go ahead now and find a mantra that allows you to embrace yourself. I love me…I am perfect…I am the best that I can be. Repeat these often and start believing them.

Speaking to Others is an Avenue to Happiness

You talk to others on a regular basis. At home, you talk to your family. At work, you talk to your employees, your bosses, and your coworkers. When you go to the grocery store, you talk to a cashier and when you go out to a restaurant, you talk to the waiter. There are social interactions happening all around you and it is important to speak to others in a positive way.

Often when you speak to others, they speak to you in a similar way. If you are tired of people talking to you in a negative way, look at how you are speaking to them before you get upset about the situation. It may be you that needs to change your ways instead of everyone else.

Be the change and person you want to see in others. If you can lead by example, it will be easier for people to follow suit. Don't expect everyone to know how to be happy and how to help you. Just as you are reading this for help, perhaps others should be as well.

Your Intonation Tells A Lot

When you talk to other people, do it in a positive way. The intonation of your voice can mean everything. It's not always what you say but how you say it. This is true even when talking to your dog. Dogs don't always understand the words you're saying but know what you're saying by the tone that you use. You can tell a dog the same words in a happy way and have him come running and say it again in a mean voice and watch him go running in the opposite direction.

Remember this as you talk to the people around you. You want to be a positive person and each time you open your mouth, you have the ability to say something nice or not so nice. How are you going to speak? Think before you speak so that you can put a positive spin on whatever is going to come out. It's hard to maintain a happy outlook all the time, but the way in which you talk to people is going to influence this heavily.

Surrounding Yourself with Happy People

One of the keys to happiness is to surround yourself with happy people. If you are always talking in a negative way to people, it's going to cause those around you to be unhappy. Misery breeds misery, which means all of you will be unhappy. Unless at least one of you can start talking in a positive way to help spread the happiness, it will take a toll on everyone.

Examples of this can be seen throughout sales and management. When a manager talks to everyone in a negative manner, this pushes everyone down instead of building them up. No one is motivated. It's not an effective way to motivate because everyone has a lower sense of self-worth after being talked to in a negative way. Sales will be down and overall productivity will be lower because everyone is wallowing in self-pity.

The moment that a manager knows how to build people up, make them feel good about themselves, and motivate them, sales will be up. Productivity will soar because everyone feels better about themselves. They have more self-confidence and are happier.

Your mood affects everyone around you. Censor yourself when talking to people so you can have a positive influence instead of a negative one. The bottom line is remembering what you can and cannot impact.

If you call a friend when you are in a negative mood, you will talk about a situation in the most negative way possible. That friend is likely going to feed your mood by helping you feel even more negative about the situation. How is that any way to get happy?

Even if a situation isn't the greatest, you can find something positive about it – or find some way to make it better. When this is the approach you use, your friend is likely going to agree with you yet again. The big revelation is that it's your mood that sets the tone for the entire conversation.

Why Beauty Pageant Contestants Do This One Thing

There are plenty of ways to approach any situation. The key is to be optimistic even when you don't want to be optimistic. If you smile, it's going to put you in a better mood. Smiling is a psychological way of tricking yourself into being happier. If you keep smiling, eventually the feeling is going to reach the rest of your body.

Women who participate in beauty pageants have learned this key quite well in their own way. They actually use Vaseline on their teeth to help them smile. If you think they are happy all the time, think again. This trick insures they are smiling when it matters most. And guess what? Within a few minutes of being forced to smile, they're in a better mood because of the action. When you go to speak to someone, you should force a smile through so you will speak in a more positive tone.

People talk to you in the same way you talk to them. If you are always doom and gloom, that's probably how people will approach you. It's hard to be positive and be happy when everyone around you is down. Someone has to be the ray of sunshine; why not you? This is your opportunity to set the tone for everyone else.

Living Around Others Means You Will Have to Forgive

When speaking with others, remember the power of forgiveness. People may do things to upset you and even though they were in the wrong, you have to be able to forgive. If you constantly hold onto a secret hatred or dislike for someone, it can eat you up inside and that's no way to be. You have to let it go and forgive. Be the bigger person and remember that everyone makes mistakes from time to time. It's not always easy to forgive, but when you can do so, it can make you feel a lot better.

Studies have been done on the power of forgiveness. When people have an attitude of forgiveness, it can lead to a higher level of heart health. This means that holding onto resentment and general dislike can actually affect your heart and forgiving can heal the heart. When you look at it like this, forgiving should definitely be at the top of your list when it comes to achieving more happiness in life.

Regardless of whether you are talking to yourself or someone else, you want to be positive. Put a positive spin on whatever you are going to say and recite some affirmations before you speak if you feel you need the extra boost of encouragement. From there, you can allow your positive mood and happiness to be contagious so that everyone around you will also be in a better mood.

Let's finish this chapter with an exercise!

Exercise 3. Create Your Own Affirmations/Incantation

1. Create an incantation or mantra where you describe yourself in a very positive manner.

2. Repeat it out loud until you memorize it and it becomes part of your identity.

3. Say your incantation every day as often as you can, including when driving, when running or when you go out for a walk.

Chapter 3
Activate Your Physiology

"It's not the strongest of the species that survives, nor the most intelligent, but the ones most responsive to change."
— Charles Darwin

Amazing Endorphin Chemicals Available to Your Brain Within Reach

You know you want to be happy, but what is it you can do in order to promote happiness? You cannot rely solely on positive thinking.

The answer is that you need to activate your physiology. The best way to do this is to get your body moving so your body produces more endorphins.

Endorphins are the magical chemicals that help make you feel good. Endorphins are responsible for locking into opioid receptors and they block the transmission of pain. They also produce a feeling of euphoria. The reason why you feel good during sex, after eating certain foods, and after exercising is because endorphins are produced during these times.

There's a physiological reason why exercising makes you feel happy. When you need a pick-me-up, the easiest thing to do is exercise, which floods the brain with more endorphins.

While you may not feel too happy while you are actually working up the sweat, the flood of endorphins will eventually occur – and when it does, this is when your brain experiences the sensation of happiness.

Endorphins Suppress Pain

The great thing about endorphins is that they act as a painkiller as well as a reward for your body. When you have hurt yourself in some way, endorphins are released to help block the pain transmission. This means you will instantly feel better because endorphins are flowing through your system.

If you have ever heard of a "runner's high", this is related to endorphins. While running, the body is suffering from oxygen. Your muscles and cells in the body are screaming for oxygen. This brings with it a euphoric feeling, and it is often why runners continue to push themselves through marathons and other competitions.

Research has shown that cardiovascular exercise as well as light to moderate weight training is capable of providing endorphins. Training that uses sprinting, heavy weights and/or anaerobic exertion are the activities that will actually produce the most endorphins – and this is the type of exercise you want to engage in to benefit in every way possible.

It's important that you understand endorphins a little bit more in depth. Endorphins are hormones that originate within the body. They are produced by the central nervous system. There are various opiates that are not produced within the body that can provide the same "high". This is why certain drugs have become popular over the years – they provide the body with a high that is similar to that of your body's own endorphins.

There is no reason to pump yourself full of illicit drugs when your body is capable of producing the happy chemicals on its own. All you need to do is understand how to activate it. When you can start moving your body and exercising in such a way that activates your physiology, you can get all the endorphins you need in order to kill pain in your body and obtain that happy feeling that you desire so much.

Produce Your Own Endorphins by Relaxing

A state of profound relaxation can produce a significant amount of endorphins. This is why it is suggested that you engage in meditation on a regular basis. When you learn how to reach a higher plane, you will feel happy because your body has produced a heavy flow of endorphins to rush through your body. This is a topic that is covered more thoroughly in its own chapter later in this book.

If you are unable to trigger enough endorphin production through exercise, or even through relaxation, acupuncture may be an option to explore as well.

Acupuncturists Use Endorphins Clinically

Clinical researchers have discovered that there are specific body acupuncture points that will produce endorphins when triggered. This way you still get the happy feeling – with the help of a practitioner.

Alternative medicine uses acupuncture for a number of reasons. It produces the endorphins without filling the body with prescription drugs, which can lead to a number of side effects. As a result, the body virtually heals itself. If you are sick or dealing with chronic pain, this is a form of alternative medicine you may want to explore to get higher levels of endorphins produced naturally within your body.

Activating Your Physiology Means Increase Your Endorphin Levels

Activating your physiology is critical so that you can experience happiness. Without endorphins flowing through your body, you will find it's difficult to experience happiness as well as to maintain it. Much of this has to do with the hormone's ability to mask pain.

Research has also shown that those who are able to release more endorphins are happier, have more positive thoughts, and are generally more optimistic as well as inspired.

There are many ways your body releases endorphins naturally. Here are a few of them:

- Laugh/smile

- Sexual intercourse

- Listening to music

- Eating spicy food

- Exercising

- Praying

- Singing

These are simple activities you can participate in but if you have denied yourself simple pleasures for a long time, it takes a bit of adjustment. By learning to simply laugh on command, it would be a lot easier to release endorphins and relieve stress.

Be open to the idea of laughing and surround yourself in a situation or environment where you can laugh easily. If you are so tense that you don't find humor in anything, even going to a comedy club won't help you laugh much but it will start the process. It's difficult to not laugh when others around you are laughing; laughter is contagious.

How Much Do You Laugh and Smile?

Remember that it's not just releasing endorphins that will help to activate your physiology. It's all about making yourself into a happier person and sometimes, this process requires a little force. Force out that smile or laugh whether you want to do so or not.

There are going to be a lot of times in life where you find yourself in a situation where you don't want to be. You have to decide right then and there how you are going to respond to it.

You could let the miserable aspects of the situation manifest and drown yourself in the dislike and hate and become more miserable as time goes on. Or you can embrace it as reality and push through it.

If you smile, there are several things that will happen.

1. You will force yourself into smiling.

2. You will show others that you are not bothered by what's going on.

3. People will gain strength from your happiness (and maybe even commend you for going with the flow.

Smiling is a sign of happiness. You may be forcing it initially, but as people smile back and you start to fake it, it will soon become something that is not forced.

It takes fewer muscles to smile than it does to frown. This means it's actually EASIER to put a smile on your face than a frown. Even if you don't want to smile and there is nothing around to smile about, it's easier to smile than frown. This means that faking it won't take too much out of you.

What Your Smile Tells Others

Once you prove to the world around you that life is not that bad and you can deal with it, you may start to believe it. The fake smile will soon turn into a real smile and that's going to lead to a higher level of happiness. It may not be the ideal situation, but you have to find something good about what's going on around you.

People may have said mean things and others may not have shown up on time for their appointment with you, but it all comes down to finding one good thing about the day, one accomplishment that was made, or something else that will help make you smile.

Have a good time in life. Love life. Smiling is easier than frowning. When you start to smile more, it will be easier to maintain a positive outlook and have a little more fun. Who cares if you don't mean what your face shows?

There's an old saying that you catch more bees with honey than vinegar, and the saying couldn't be truer within life. If someone tells a joke, don't be a stick in the mud. Just laugh about it and have fun with it.

Smile. Smiling is a universal sign you are happy and it makes you more approachable. It can help you with life in general. Your boss may be more likely to give you a raise when you smile and people are more likely to approach you in social situations when you have a smile on your face.

Go ahead and give it a try. The next time life is not going your way, activate your physiology and change things around a little bit differently. Smile. Put a big smile on your face and see how it will make you feel. As a smile tugs on the muscles of your face, it may give you a false sense that everything is good with the world. When people see the smile on your face, they may find you to be more of a happy-go-lucky person – and you may win some new friends.

Smiling is a feel good action. As Yoko Ono once said, "Smile in the mirror. Do that every morning and you'll start to see a big difference in your life." These are definitely words to live by. If you don't believe it, go ahead and do it each morning for a week. You will start to see improvements within your life, including a higher level of happiness.

Have More Sex

All your problems won't be solved by sex, but some of them may be solved with it. Sex can be a lot of fun, especially when you're with the right partner. It's a way of connecting with someone you have feelings for and when you reach the pinnacle, the rush of hormones, adrenaline and serotonin leaves you satiated on a higher level. Sexual intercourse can relieve stress, making you a happier person.

Going too long without sex once you have had it the first time can leave you feeling stressed and frustrated. This is why there are sex therapists, marriage counselors, and sex consultants to work with. If you're unable to have sex with your partner, then you may be much less happier than you could be – and it's going to affect your mood in a variety of negative ways.

Sex is a healthy part of any stable relationship and you feel good when you have it. This means that you should actually have it with frequency so you can experience the rush of hormones that keeps you happy.

Go ahead and tell your partner you would like to have some more of it. It can be great for both of you. If you're in a committed relationship, it may be exactly the release you need – and the happiness that comes from it can impact your life in a variety of positive ways.

Listen to Music to Boost Those Endorphins

Listening to music or singing can be one of the most powerful ways to release endorphins and achieve happiness. Music provides two sensations, not one – audio and tactile. The audio can help to tune the rest of the world out so you can focus solely on the beat and the music. You can lose yourself in the lyrics and the overall sensation of music.

Music is also tactile when it's loud enough. The bass can help to vibrate through your body and help calm you. It can help unlock something within your body and hum you into a quieter place, similar to that of meditation.

Various types of music can affect your mood. If you go into a gym, you'll never hear soft piano instrumentals because it keeps people too calm. Instead, the music is hard hitting beats and techno that help to get the endorphins going and keep people moving around. People are happy at the gym and they're able to get a good workout in – and some of this has to do with the music that's being piped in.

When you want to activate your physiology, sometimes the answer is music. Listen to music. Listen to loud music. And listen to music that makes you happy.

When the music doesn't work, you can turn to some of the other things on the list, such as sex, or chili peppers, or something else.

Use Your Senses to Boost Your Endorphins

Your daily life is full of sensory input. Your nose smells aromas, your fingers touch objects, your mouth feels textures, your taste buds taste foods, your ears hear sounds and your eyes see. As you embrace all these senses, you can activate your physiology and improve your mood. Some people respond better by using one sense over another one, so spend a little time determining which sense channel works best for you.

Some people need chocolate and other foods to calm them down and unlock various parts of their emotions. This would mean their predominant sense channel that brings them happiness is the sense of taste.

Other people respond better with smell. Aromatherapy in particular can be effective. Various essential oils are great for engaging the sense of smell and have an impact on how you feel. Lavender essential oil is calming. Citrus is stimulating and eucalyptus can be therapeutic in that it opens up the nasal passageways and leads to healing congestion there.

It is beneficial to look at various images that are soothing to your mind. Now, you can do this in many ways, not only going to the forest or on a mountain walk. There are light sensory helmets you can strap onto your head that provide a unique sensory experience. You can also walk through an art gallery. Get creative and experiment with what you can do to provide soothing images because you never know what's going to work best for you.

Why Not Have More Fun in Your Life?

Embrace the fun in life! When you have fun, it can help you to forget about the stress of the world and it can activate more of your physiology. Go for the adrenaline rush with roller coasters or base jumping or get out of the house and play a round of golf. Doing something you enjoy can fulfill a basic need at the core of your being for experiencing variation – and make it easier to feel joy on a regular basis.

If you don't already have a hobby, it can be a good idea to develop one. Follow a sports team, learn how to draw, play a game, or choose something else. Whether it's you alone or participating in sports with a group of friends, it can be exactly what you need to relax, have a good time and release more endorphins.

Eat Spicy Food and Boost Your Metabolism and Serotonin

Spicy food is capable of providing benefits to your body and your emotions. Whether it's chili, hot sauce, or some other spicy food, think about incorporating more spicy food into your diet from time to time. Health benefits include boosting your metabolism and lowering blood pressure.

Too much stress raises your blood pressure if you can't deal with the stress. If you can counteract some stress with spicy salsa, hot wings, or a spicy

Thai dish, it's to your advantage to do so. You can add years to your life and be a happier person throughout those added years.

The spiciness is also going to help raise levels of the feel-good hormones, including serotonin. It's always helpful to have more of these flowing through your body, so if it means asking for the spicier version of something the next time you go to a restaurant, then go ahead and order it up. It will ease the feelings of stress and depression and bring a smile to your face, even if it brings a tear to your eye at the same time!

Count on Exercise to Give You Many Benefits

Exercise is capable of giving you more energy, more oxygen to the brain, and many other benefits. Whether it's a run, a trip to the gym, or a swim in the pool, working your muscles activates your physiology on a whole new level. Fifteen percent of all cardiac output goes to the brain and that will help improve your memory, your thinking processes and decision-making ability, and much more.

When you exercise regularly, your body will build up less lactic acid in the muscles. The accumulation of the lactic acid in the muscles is what causes fatigue. This means if you're feeling a little sleepy (which can lead to depression), the best thing you can do is get up and move around!

Since the age of 14, I have practiced sports whenever possible. I played Ice hockey for several years until I went to University, and I remember telling myself that I would run, swim, bike, skate or go to the gym for the rest of my life.

When I was 30, I ran so often that I decided to apply for the NYC marathon, which I did in 1999 and 2000! Running was my favorite way to feel good, reduce stress, relax and produce my endorphin dosages.

Today, I am in my mid 40's and still work out 3 to 5 times a week. Mother Nature gave you legs, arms and a brain; this is all you need to run, swim, bike or just move, and as a result, you will feel good.

But why do so many people procrastinate on this, prefer to sit on couch, eat snacks drink sodas and watch TV? Well, it's more comfortable to be lazy and to stay in your comfort zone. However, if you want to feel strong, be happier, have a lean body, and have more endurance in your life, working out on a daily basis will help you. I recently read a scientific study showing that people training for endurance can deal better with stress and pressure than those who don't.

Additional Benefits of Activating Your Physiology

In some instances, you may need to create actionable goals in order to achieve the benefits mentioned above. Releasing endorphins is easy but you may need to work at it a little bit at first. For example, if you want to have more sex, you may need to first find a partner or you may need to work out some issues with your current partner. Things like eating spicier food and listening to music are easier – and therefore, you may want to start with these.

Throughout some of the next chapters, you will learn about meditation and yoga, which can help you transcend your normal brain activity and slow brain activity down so that you are not consumed by thought and external stimuli.

As you begin to relax, you can engage in all these different activities. Sex with your partner can be exciting, invigorating, and relaxing at the same time. Endorphins are going to flood your system, allowing you to forget some of the pain that you have as well as to excite you in a new way.

Every one of these activities can provide you with the release of endorphins that you need. Your body can begin to heal and you can begin to let all the stress of your day slip away.

Even socializing can help your body produce more endorphins. If you've ever felt strangely excited after meeting a stranger, it is because your body has produced endorphins. If you have ever noticed that social people are happier, this is the reason for it. Those who tend to be antisocial often suffer from depression – and one of the main reasons is because they have not activated their physiology effectively to produce enough endorphins to be happy and have a high level of well being.

Use Variation During the Day to Keep You Going

It's a good idea to change things up a bit to experience various forms of stimuli that will release endorphins. While you may want to have sex every day, it may not be something that is possible. This means you should plan on experiencing different stimuli.

Buy tickets to a comedy club or get a gym membership. Find a new Spanish restaurant in town that is known for having spicy food or go to a rock concert. By changing things up a bit, you will ensure that you have fun, relaxed, and develop a higher level of happiness.

Being social is important and when you can have more fun throughout the week, it is a guarantee that you will be able to relieve some stress out of your life. Being able to release stress is critical to your ability to not only release endorphins, but also achieve happiness. If you are too high strung as a result of stress in your life, it will be impossible for you to let go long enough to experience happiness in any capacity.

Endorphins not only make you happy but also help you relax. This means that you can eliminate a lot of stress by having more endorphins course through your body. It doesn't matter whether you get the endorphins through exercise or through food. You want to be less depressed, less anxious, and less stressed. It has been proven that this brain chemical is capable of helping you achieve all these things, so you are going to be happier and healthier for it.

Choose to Boost Your Endorphins Daily

Throughout this book, the things you are learning will allow you to better control your emotions and attract positive events in your life. There are various things you can do just by making better choices in your life. Endorphins are an important part of your life and now you know why. It isn't something you can "hope" for; it's actual cause and effect. You can take action to produce endorphins on your own so you are in control of your overall mood and emotions.

Now that you know why endorphins are important to your ability to become happy and how to get your body to produce them, start activating their production as often as possible. You don't always have to exercise and you don't always have to be social. However, when you can find the balance so that you produce these hormonal miracles in one way or another on a daily basis, you can always have a smile and a positive way of thinking.

There are some added benefits of boosting your physiology as well. Once you get the flow of endorphins going, you won't just relax and become a happier person. Medical research confirms through exercise physiology that unlocking your physiology and journaling can help you recover from a variety of health conditions.

Learning how to get endorphins flowing through the body has helped people with diabetes, PTSD, chronic pain, arthritis, osteoporosis, and even cancer.

Choose Exercise That Fits You

Exercise does not always have positive effects on the musculoskeletal system, which is why you need to work with various other methods of releasing endorphins. Your doctor can talk to you about exercises that will work for your level of fitness or rehabilitation.

When you do not want to exercise or are not able to exercise to the level that you want, there are still plenty of other activities that will boost your physiology. You can choose yoga, which is easy on the joints and provides a deep level of relaxation so that you can reap benefits in other ways as well.

You Can Control Your Physiology

Your physiology is not something that should be ignored. Knowing how to control your physiology can help with muscle strength and endurance, flexibility, and brings mental and physical benefits. When you have a strong body both mentally and physically, you can enjoy life to the fullest because you will be able to do all the things that you want to do without being limited in any capacity.

Essentially, boosting your physiology is a matter of getting up and doing things. Moping around the house and feeling sorry for yourself for extended periods of time does not work. It is not healthy and leads to depression. When you boost your physiology, you become active and this allows you to get more things done.

Your body runs more efficiently when you have boosted your physiology. Whenever your body meets resistance, it is not running efficiently and this means you are using more energy than what is necessary. Your entire body requires energy in order to function.

If your body is spending too much energy dealing with health conditions, you won't have energy for other things. As a result, you need to make sure that you have unlocked your physiology completely so your body runs more effectively and you have the energy needed to do everything you want to do.

What Will You Do With More Energy?

Having more energy can allow you to get more things done. You will be able to see how more things can get accomplished and how you can reach more than one goal at a time because you have the energy to get it all done. Some of the simplest things in life require energy, and if your body is running efficiently, less energy is needed for breathing, heart rate and blood pressure, allowing more energy to be available for the other things going on in your life.

Having more vitality and energy allows you to accomplish more during your day, and this is something everyone should desire. It is even more important if you have a family with children, because you will have more time for them. We are all so busy in our life, working one or more jobs, doing daily responsibilities, and trying to have fun all at the same time. Imagine waking up every morning, jumping out of bed and feeling strong and happy. How would you feel?

This emotional state can be achieved, though it requires discipline, commitment and willpower. There are only 24 hours in a day, but you can make the most out of each of those 24 hours so you begin to live the life you want.

Exercise 4. Create Your Endorphin-Building Activity List

1. Think of several different activities that will increase your endorphin levels. Will you go to the gym every day? Meditate? Sing? Spend more time making love with your partner more often?

2. Write down your plan for the next 30 days.

3. Practice!

Chapter 4
The Socialization Factor

We Wither Away Without Others

Socializing is an important part of being happy. If you analyze hermits, you would find them in a state of fear and depression.

Hermits are clueless about what's going on in the real world and for whatever reason, are missing a huge part of what it is to be human. We are pack animals by nature and thrive when we have friends who can be a part of our ups and downs.

You Can Choose Your Level of Socialization

It doesn't matter whether you're an introvert or an extrovert. The key is to socialize at a level that you feel comfortable with and fits a basic need. You will feel confident with the group that you interact with and there's no need to do a lot of socializing if you don't feel comfortable. Some people need daily interactions while others need it weekly or monthly. Identify what you need and then be sure to seek it out.

With social media and the Internet, it is easier to get the socialization factor more than ever before. You can chat with people online all day long and never meet up with them face to face. If you are a private person or don't make friends easily, this is a great way to continue socializing at a level that brings you happiness.

Socialization Means Support Groups

When you spend time with a group of people, whether it is online or face-to-face, you can have a support group. These are people who are going to sense that you are down without you having to say anything. They can lift your mood – and you can do the same for them when they are down.

Sometimes it is hard to get the help you need on your own. You cannot always look at the bright side. You need someone to point it out and help find it. This is why it's important to have friends around. Those whispers of encouragement may be just what are needed to make it through the day or week. If you don't have anyone whispering words of encouragement, it could lead to depression because there's no one around to pull you out of the darkness that comes from time to time – and that's a scary place to be.

With reminders of how much you are loved and adored, you can prevent slipping into the darkness. Just as you need words of affirmation to remind yourself how great you are, you need words of affirmation from others as well. It's not selfish or egotistical. It is part of the human experience – and one you shouldn't hesitate to find in one way or another.

Facebook Fulfills a Need

A Facebook account connects you with friends and is a great way to socialize and get some encouragement. Whether you talk to those people on a regular basis or not, you can rely on at least some of them to be there for you in your time of need.

Go ahead and perform an experiment with your Facebook account. The next time you're feeling down, post a message. Watch how many people respond and give you uplifting messages. It is a way to counteract the negative in your life and find the positive. It's important to find happiness and whether you realize it or not, there are people out there who are there to help you find it. Sometimes it just takes a little bit of a prompt to get people to realize where you're at and what kind of help you need.

Have You Ever Noticed Different Levels of Socialization Exist?

There are different levels of socialization and each one is important to you and your overall level of happiness. The different levels are family, friends, peer groups, and co-workers. Each of these levels need friends and when people are missing from one or more groups, it shows what you need to work on.

Your family is going to love you unconditionally. They may live near or far, but they will be there for you through the hardest parts of your life.

Reaching out to them should be done with some frequency, as they may be able to help you on a very primitive level of your being because of the blood bond that is shared. In some instances, there is no family where you share a blood bond, but you have a bond over shared experiences, tragedies, or struggles – and these people can be considered family as well.

Choose Your Friends Wisely

Your friends are ones you have chosen to be in your life and it's likely because they share similarities in the thinking patterns as well as shared interests. When people share your thinking patterns and interests, it's a huge plus because they can help with decision making and provide socialization when you want to get out of the house and have some fun. These are likely the people you are going to spend the most time with – and it's critical that you make time for them so you can get what you need.

Don't Ignore Peer Group Friends

Your peer groups are acquaintances that may be around you because of shared hobbies and interests. If you go to the gym, there are going to be people you see on a regular basis and while you may not get together with them outside of the gym, they are your friends while there.

Developing more conversation between these groups can be important, as it will allow you to enjoy yourself more. You can have someone to talk to, someone to encourage and push you, and you will have people you can look after as well. Some of the peer groups may have individuals within them who are in need of tutoring and/or guidance. Deciding to take on this role and a nurturing aspect can lead to happiness within your life because it is an unselfish act.

It's Wise to Get Along with People at Work

Finally, you have your co-workers on another level. It's important to be friendly to this group because they are going to be with you every day. You may actually see and interact with these people more than everyone else.

At a job, it's very possible you will see these people eight hours a day, five days a week. If you don't get along with your co-workers, it can turn a day into a very long and boring existence – and possibly a frustrated one if you are at each other's throats.

While it's not easy to get along with everyone, you should be focusing on ways to make it tolerable and open up the line of communication. If you can get along with your co-workers, it will be easier to find happiness – and they will be happier about the situation as well.

Socialization is Many Things

Socialization happens on so many levels and it needs to be considered and worked on. Having people in your life that you are close to, get along with, and who understand you is critical to your happiness.

If you are not happy, those are the people who will cheer you up. You may have noticed already that cheering up each other becomes the task of the group – and the person needing cheering up changes all the time. This is how you work together to achieve happiness. You may be the happy one in the group this week and it is your responsibility to spread the cheer – and the following week it may be someone else's turn to do it to you.

How Many Selfish People are In Your Life?

You cannot hang out with selfish people for too long. If you find that you are always providing emotional support for your friends but they cannot return the favor, they are not true friends. Think about finding new friends.

It is not always easy to sever ties with "friends", but if your happiness is on the line, it may be the only true way to find the happiness you long for. You need friends who give and take. If all they do is take, it is a one-sided relationship and one you are not benefitting from in any capacity.

You Can Improve Your Socialization Skills No Matter What Age You Are

It's okay if socializing isn't something you're particularly good at. As with some of the other concepts within this book, the first step is to identify what is an issue. From there, you can work on it with more frequency so your basic need is met. It may not be easy and may require you to step out from your comfort zone from time to time.

Remember that socialization can occur from inside your home, on the computer, at work, when you're out with friends, and anywhere else you go. Explore various methods because you will find that you likely need to use a little bit of all of them in order to meet your needs.

Introverts and extroverts alike can socialize and be happy; find the balance that allows you to be happy. Sometimes it means going out with friends even when you don't want to or joining a social club as a way of meeting like-minded individuals.

Do what you have to do in order to find happiness. Once you have a good balance of people in your life and everyone takes turns feeding into each other's needs and wants, it is easier to find happiness and hold onto it for longer periods of time because the socialization factor has been taken care of.

Exercise 5. Who Has Motivated and Inspired You?

1. Make a List of all your friends, family members, and business partners that have inspired you. Which ones have kept you motivated in the past?

2. Send these people a note or call them, telling them how important they have been for you in your life, and say thank you.

Chapter 5
The Physiological Effects of Unhappiness

"If you do what you love, it is the best way to relax."
— *Christian Louboutin*

Being Unhappy Brings Negative Physiological Changes

There are many physiological effects of unhappiness. Sometimes you need a reason to be happy. Do you think that happiness is a big deal? Do you think happiness is overrated? If so, reconsider these thoughts with information presented in this chapter. By learning about the physiological effects of unhappiness, you quickly find out why it's not where you want to be for long.

Your body functions better when it is happy. A happy body equals a happy you. When your body becomes unhappy, unpleasant things happen – and you may not be aware of all of them. Your unhappiness can lead to depression and stress, not just for you but also for the people around you. Your unhappiness can be toxic to those who have to live with you. If you don't want to get happy, think about what your unhappiness is doing to those you love most in life.

Your unhappiness can also weaken your body, leaving you sick more often. Unhappiness may be the very thing that causes a shorter life. Consider that for a moment. If you continue to be unhappy, it can reduce your life expectancy. If you want to live a long and healthy life, figure out how to turn your unhappiness around.

Unhappiness and stress are closely linked. Stress can be felt in your arms, legs and joints and affect how you function. To put it simply, unhappiness and stress are not good for your body. This means that you want to avoid them whenever possible so you can have a more exciting and more fulfilling life – and ensure that others in your life are able to do the same. Remember that you control whether you are unhappy or not – just flip the switch to change the emotions you experience.

Side Effects of Stress: Have You Found Them?

There are countless side effects of stress and generally, it is not good for you. While some people say they thrive on stress, this statement is only partially true. Stress will hit a breaking point where people have too much of it. At that point, the body is no longer able to deal with stress positively. This is when the negative side effects of stress are seen and felt.

Stress can impact the amount of sleep you get and the quality of the sleep once you are able to fall asleep. It can give you a less than peaceful night of sleep because you are lying in bed thinking about everything that you're not getting done or that you're upset about. Insomnia and other sleep problems appear as a result of being too stressed.

Too much stress or stress handled poorly will weaken your immune system. If you have ever noticed you seem to get sick every time you are run down and have a million and one things on your plate, it's because you have weakened your immune system and basically allowed yourself to get sick because you weren't taking care of yourself. When you are especially stressed, it's also hard to recover from any illness. Your body's way of slowing you down and showing you to change priorities is to make you sick.

Stress Can Immobilize You

Stress can literally weigh you down and make it hard to move. It creates tension in your muscles and when you wake up one morning, you may find it hard to get out of bed and walk across the room. This is going to have an impact on how you feel and how you get motivated to get things done. With too much stress, everything is a struggle and takes longer when you are in physical pain. Why be in pain when you have the ability not to be?

Learning to let go and find an outlet for stress can be one of the healthiest things you can do for yourself. This idea returns us to the thought of how important it is to make sure your body is running as efficiently as possible.

Worst Case Scenario: Stress Prevents the Next Generation from Emerging

Did you know that chronic stress could also lead to infertility in both men and women? Women stop ovulating when they have high levels of stress and men may deal with erectile dysfunction or a low sperm count. This means you are doing yourself a huge injustice by staying stressed – how can you create the family you want to be able to create in the future?

Stress Brings On Serious Illnesses

Stress also raises your blood pressure through the release of hormones such as cortisol and adrenaline pumping through your system. With high levels of these hormones, you are at a higher risk for health problems such as stroke, kidney failure, heart attack, and even blindness.

These should all be eye-opening reasons why you need to reduce some of the stress in your life. Some stress is good because it can allow you to remain focused on the task at hand. Too much stress, however, is bad for the body and bad for everyone around you. It's not normal to feel so stressed that you feel like you could burst at any situation.

The ways you deal with stress depend upon what you are faced with on a day-to-day basis. Some stress can be dealt with physically while some has to be dealt with emotionally. One thing is for sure – too much stress in your life is not going to allow you to be happy. You don't want to be toxic to yourself or to others, so it is in your best interest to learn how to deal with the stress. Eliminate it or at least greatly reduce it.

Understanding Cortisol and What it Does

Cortisol is a hormone secreted by the adrenal glands of your body. If you want to be happy and healthy, learn what you can about cortisol. You need this hormone flowing through your body because it helps metabolize glucose, enhances immunity, lowers the inflammatory response, and even regulates your blood pressure.

Cortisol is Good or Bad Depending on the Amount Released

Small increases of cortisol will give you a boost of energy, enhance your memory, reduce your sensitivity to pain, and even maintain the homeostasis for day-by-day survival. Too much cortisol in your body at any given time and for prolonged periods however is bad.

You Can Order a Cortisol Test Yourself

It's good to find out what your levels of cortisol are. There are places online where you can order a cortisol test such as www.LEF.org, the Life Extension Foundation. You don't need a doctor's prescription to order this test. Knowing your cortisol levels tells you exactly whether or not your body is producing it when necessary and if the levels are in check throughout the day.

Doctors call cortisol the stress hormone because it is secreted in higher levels when you are stressed. Too much stress means too much cortisol and that's not healthy.

High Cortisol? Reducing Your Stress is the Simplest Solution

What can you do about it? The easiest way to ensure that your levels are not too high is to not let your body get too stressed. This sounds easier to say than do but there are ways to reduce the stress in your life – and your body will be better for it.

Why is cortisol such a bad thing? Before you can start to reduce cortisol, you have to know why it's a problem. Here's a long list of why high levels are bad and why reducing your stress levels should be a priority:

- Decreases bone density

- Impairs cognitive skills

- Suppresses thyroid function

- Decreases muscle tissue

- Causes blood sugar imbalances

- Lowers immune function

- Increases abdominal fat

- Causes erectile dysfunction

You Get to Choose How You Experience Life's Moments

Just as you can experience a situation as a stressor, you can also relax and thus reduce your cortisol levels. Stress activates the fight or flight mode of the nervous system. A big rush of cortisol gives you the energy and tools needed to fight your opposition, but then you must be able to relax and essentially recover from what has happened.

If you don't give your body the relaxation time it's waiting for, the cortisol will continue to be produced. That's when you end up having negative side effects.

Time to Be Honest About Your Stress and Cortisol Levels

To help you better understand why cortisol can be such a bad thing, go back through and look at the list of negative results from it above. How many of them did you have? Who needs a number of health problems from excessive amounts of cortisol?

You are literally weakening your body because of the chronic stress and ends up costing you more in doctor visits, prescription drugs, and time away from work, which will likely cause you more stress. What really is happening here is the creation of a vicious circle that's difficult to break, all because of the feeling of being stressed.

The increase in abdominal fat is not a good or fun thing to experience either. Many people with chronic stress have a significant amount of excess belly fat. This is directly related to the cortisol and as long as your body continues producing the cortisol, this fat will remain. Working out at the gym every day still won't eliminate it. The bottom line is if you don't deal with the stress, not only will you see more fat but soon your muscle tissue will appear to be dwindling.

Belly fat is likely to cause self-esteem issues because you don't look as good as you want to and as good as you know you could. Low self-esteem may lead to low self-confidence. Low self-confidence leads to an array of other negative emotions because you don't feel motivated, creative, and happy.

Your health and your happiness are defined by the very things that cortisol can destroy. You really have no choice but to keep the hormone in check – and the primary way to do that is by reducing the amount of stress in your life.

Regardless of how much cortisol and stress you have invited into your life up to this point, you can make the decision to change some things. Cortisol is lowered when you reduce the stress so there is no time like the present to start reducing the stress in your life. You'll end up with more control over your emotions and invite better, healthier emotions into your life.

How to Rid the Body of Stress

Now it's time to learn how to eliminate stress. Stress cannot be eliminated with the simple flip of a switch, so you have to be more active at reducing and eliminating stresses from your life. Some stress is good. However, when it reaches the point of chronic stress and affects your body negatively, it's time to raise your hand and start asking for some help in eliminating it.

7 Ways to Eliminate Stress and Lower Cortisol

Everyone has their own method of eliminating stress and your methods may even change over the years. What works for someone else may not work for you – at least not at first. Below is a list of various ways to eliminate stress – and even prevent stress from entering your life to begin with.

1. Meditate or pray.

>Inhale and exhale slowly. "Feel" the bad air leaving and good air entering. There are various books and even apps you can get to help you with some guided breathing exercises. (Give examples)

2. Drink a cup of black tea.

>Black tea is not only delicious but also may help you deal with stress and lower your cortisol. Drink it either hot or cold. Did you know that black tea offers other benefits, too? Since your stress level falls, you may find your libido levels rising. Lower blood pressure and an overall better outlook on life also are quite common.

3. Practice yoga.

>Yoga offers an array of health benefits and reducing stress is one of them. Many people swear by yoga when it comes to living a happier life. You don't need to go to a yoga studio to practice yoga; try it at home or at work. Striking a few yoga poses may help re-align you by making you slow down, thus dissipating the stress quickly.

4. Play sports.

>Any sport will get you moving and release some aggression. Each time you whack a ball with a tennis racquet, a baseball bat, or even your hand, you can pretend it is something that is affecting your life. Competitive sports is also great for reducing stress levels even more because it adds an extra social factor to your life.

5. Aromatherapy.

>Scents affect your mood. Lavender is one of the most calming scents and it is known to lower stress-related chemicals, such as cortisol. You can light a lavender candle, put a few drops of lavender essential oil near you, or even use a body lotion infused with the scent.

6. Take a vacation.

Taking a vacation is not running away from your problems; it's reducing your stress levels. Vacations allow you to rest and recharge so you will go back to your job and life with more energy and even a new approach – all without stress.

7. Get a pet.

Having a furry friend or pet to come home to allow you to turn your head off. Your pet is your instant buddy to curl up with on the coach, talk to, and go for long walks with. And petting a pet has long been known for lowering blood pressure and heart rate. What a great way to de-stress after a long day at the office! Pets prevent you from taking out your problems on loved ones.

Foods Fighting the Battle of Depression

What are your best ways to fight depression? While all the ideas previously presented may help, there's one major area to look at to fight depression: your diet.

Some foods are naturally better at fighting stress than others – and it's advantageous to work them into your diet.

6 Foods That Fight Depression

Here's a list of 6 foods that can change your moods:

1. Turkey

Turkey contains the amino acid tryptophan, which is known to stimulate serotonin in the brain. Serotonin is a neurotransmitter that gives you a feel-good vibe.

2. Walnuts

Walnuts fight depression because they contain omega 3-fatty acids, which support brain health.

3. Low-fat Dairy Products

Whether it's a glass of milk, a cup of yogurt, or even low-fat cheese, dairy products have a good amount of protein and vitamin D, which will fight depression. One cup of milk gives you about 12 grams protein. Milk can also help you feel relaxed.

4. Whole grains

Whole grains include whole wheat, oats, rye, rice, amaranth, spelt, corn and quinoa. Any of these foods may be eaten as cereal or mixed with other foods to make salads or even desserts. One little-known fact about whole grains is that serotonin is released when you eat them. Thus, if you're eating whole grains, you're managing your stress levels.

5. Turmeric

This boldly yellow spice is curry. By adding it to any of your dishes such as grains with vegetables, stir-fry and rice dishes, you may find that your mood lifts. Turmeric is also an inflammation-buster and a stress reducer. It's no wonder that people who own Indian restaurants are so happy! If you never believed in the spice of life, start believing.

6. Vitamin C

Take a Vitamin C supplement, 500 to 1000 mg a day. People who have high levels of vitamin C do not show the expected mental and physical signs of stress when subjected to acute psychological challenges. What's more, they bounce back from stressful situations faster than people with low levels of vitamin C in their blood.

There are many other foods and supplements as well but start with these. Familiarize yourself with them and take advantage of their benefits of reducing stress. Set a goal of eating one of these daily; then increase it later to higher amounts.

Beating the Stress

Stress doesn't need to be an everyday part of life. You will be happier when there is less stress around you. Don't ever expect it to be possible that you will remove stress from your life entirely.

However, there are always ways you can think of that will eliminate stress. This way, the stress that remains won't weigh on your shoulders and take a toll on you physiologically.

What Emotions Are You Choosing During Your Day?

Happiness and health are greatly impacted by your emotions and their effect on your physiology. Something as simple as too much stress can weaken your immune system and cause you to get sick with greater frequency. The good news is that there are various choices you can make to control the stress that you deal with on a daily basis.

One thing to remember is that you need to stay tuned into your body so that you can recognize when you reach the level of stress that is unmanageable. Having people close to you who help you identify when you are stressed can help you as well. Keep your stress in check and watch how easy it is to be happier, healthier, and generally enjoy life throughout the years.

Exercise 6. Commit to Lowering Your Stress Levels Today

1. Make a decision and commitment right now to lower your stress.

2. Create a plan on how you can choose one or two things every day that will lower stress. For example, instead of drinking your daily coffee, switch to green tea or black tea. Work out or exercise on a regular basis, 2 to 3 times a week or more.

3. Write a weekly plan and be disciplined.

4. Stick to your plan for at least six weeks.

Chapter 6
Remove the Poisons

"Success consists of going from failure to failure without
loss of enthusiasm."
— Winston Churcill

Foods Either Nourish You or They Don't

You are what you eat. Just as there are foods you should eat because they make you feel amazing and help you to feel the best that you can feel, there are foods that do the very opposite. These should be known as poisons.

You consume poisons every day. We're not talking about anything radioactive or something that comes with a warning label and is stored underneath your kitchen sink. There are poisons you put into your body that slow you down, destroy your organs, and make you unhealthy.

By identifying these poisons, you position yourself to make healthier decisions about what you eat and drink. You can choose not to eat the poison. There are thousands of foods to choose from; why not choose better foods that can feed your body? The problem is that most people have no idea what they are eating that is so bad for them.

Poisons Can Be Counted On to Affect Your Moods

Some of the poisons that go into your body affect your mood. There are literally foods you eat that can cause mood swings. What we're talking about here goes beyond being an emotional eater. Some foods can cause a spike in your blood sugar so you are suddenly angry, tired, feeling stressed, or depressed.

Why would you put any of these foods in your body if you could avoid them? You could be eating foods right now that are causing you to stress out even further or lash out at your loved ones.

Do You Poison Your Moods With What You Eat?

Poisoning your mood is the worst thing you can do, and you are doing it without even knowing. Think about it. Do you want to keep eating foods that prevent you from achieving happiness? No matter how good the food may taste, you need to use your mind and understand how it can be affecting those around you.

Insight Into Addicts Behavior

When it comes to alcohol and drug abuse, the first step is awareness. Addicts need to be able to identify that they are addicts because that is the pathway to finding help. The same can be true about poison consumption. Accept that there is a problem and then make the choice to get the help and cut them out of your life.

You don't need highs and lows within your day because it makes you unpredictable. Those close to you may know that if you eat a certain food, they have to keep their distance from you for the rest of the afternoon because you are irritable. Who wants to be the bear at the office or at the house that everyone wants to avoid? It's not going to make you any friends.

When you learn about the poisons and how they affect you, it's easier to eliminate them from your diet so you can put better things into your body. Eliminating them allows you to reach a better balance of emotions, have a more positive influence on those around you, and develop better relationships with coworkers, family members, and friends.

Get Rid of the Poisons By Cleaning Up Your Diet

The poisons may be hiding in foods you eat or they may be blatantly there for you to see, and you choose to eat them anyway. By choosing to remove the poisons, you improve your health.

Some of the poisons that are consumed daily include:

- Alcohol

- Coffee

- Sugar

- Meat

- Dairy

- Trans fats

If you look at this list, you may be wondering if there is any food left that you can eat. The answer is yes, absolutely. Some foods on this list can still be eaten, but in smaller quantities.

Some poisons also hide in foods you love. Sugar is often hidden in a variety of different foods that are available to eat – even when you try to avoid it.

A Special Note About Meat and Dairy Foods

You may be able to live without alcohol or trans fats, but what about meat and dairy? You don't have to eliminate all foods on the list but you consider reducing their intake, especially if you have been suffering from health problems as a result of ingesting them. Many people lack the enzymes required to digest all these foods and it can literally make them sick.

What About Alcohol and Coffee?

Alcohol shouldn't require any kind of list of reasons as to why it is on the list. Alcohol is addictive, reduces your reaction time and can contribute to mistakes while driving, and even damage your liver if you drink to excess on occasion. That's not to say you can never have alcohol again. Be smart about when you drink it and how much you have of it you have during one sitting.

Coffee is another one of those foods that should be limited. It may be what you use to wake up in the morning because of the caffeine rush delivered to your system. Part of what's so bad about coffee is all of the cream and sugar that is dumped into it. If you drink your coffee black, it will make it easier to remove some of the poisons from your daily routine.

There are many reasons as to why you may want to quit drinking coffee.

1. Coffee increases your stress hormone cortisol.

2. Coffee decreases your sensitivity to insulin

3. Drinking coffee can result in addiction.

4. Coffee has a high level of acidity, which is why your stomach may be grumbling after you drink it.

If you really love the pick-me-up that coffee offers, consider some alternatives for the pick-me-up feeling. Some examples include tea, caffeine-free herbal coffee (chicory or dandelion root), yerba mate, periwinkle tea or even wheatgrass juice. These are easier to digest and will provide you with the energy boost needed in the morning or in the middle of the day.

Why Is Sugar So Bad When It Tastes So Good?

Sugar is found in many foods. Once you identify it on the label, make better food selections so you don't eat sugar without knowing it. It hurts your teeth as well as the rest of your body. Sugar is famous for its "empty" calories, and that's never a good thing for your body – or your waistline. Empty calories mean calories without any nutrients. Foods with empty calories end up robbing the nutrients from your body stores because they have no nutrients of their own.

Some other reasons you may want to reduce the amount of sugar in your diet include overloading your liver with work, insulin resistance, diabetes, cancer, and other degenerative health problems.

Limit Excess Fat With Food Choices

Meat and dairy products aren't poisons if you choose the better choices in these categories. Lean is always the way to go because you can avoid putting more fat in your body than what is necessary. Portion control is also an important aspect with both meat and dairy. Eating an abundance of these foods means you are taking in higher calorie counts plus you are also experiencing their effects they have on your digestive system.

What About Trans Fats?

The next poison to avoid is trans fats. These are considered the worst fats because they are created during a hydrogenation process. Hydrogenated fats lurk in almost all processed foods such as cookies and French fries at your favorite fast food restaurant.

These used to be hidden fats but by law, they must be identified now. Become more aware of what's in your foods by reading the labels before you place them in your cart.

Reducing Food Poisons Is Critical to Your Happiness

While these foods are poisons, it doesn't mean you have to avoid all of them all of the time. Be more aware of what they are capable of doing to harm you so you can control the overall consumption of them.

This means you can still have a cup of coffee in the morning – but be aware of what it can do. You may also want to consider substituting green tea for the coffee out periodically. You get more health benefits and your emotions stay stable with green tea. You can still have a glass of wine at night or even a martini out with friends as long as you don't drink to excess.

The poisons are found all day long. From the moment you wake up, you are faced with various poisons you can choose to put into your body – and those temptations continue throughout the day. When you have identified the poisons and mastered how to eliminate them, substituted them for healthier foods, or managed them in an effective manner, you boost your positive flow of energy and are a happier person to be around.

My Personal Story About Coffee Addiction

I used to be a coffee junky, drinking 8 to 10 cups a day, every day, even on Sunday! I was always nervous, anxious and irritable. It was difficult for me to focus on tasks and I gained weight that was hard to lose. I remember the day I decided to quit drinking coffee.

I made a commitment to my family, my mentor, and myself. The withdrawal symptoms lasted five days, and then came the big revelation. I realized how coffee was controlling my mind. Coffee was a poison, not a food because you don't get withdrawal symptoms from a food! Coffee is an addictive drug.

I was poisoning myself with an edible drug that was available on the market and hadn't even known it until I quit. Now I drink plenty of green tea and sometimes black tea with a squeezed lemon, and the quality of my life increased so much. I sleep better, I am more focused, work more efficiently and productively, wake up in the morning very easily without any need of coffee to keep me going.

I absolutely recommend lowering your coffee consumption, and if you're brave and want to raise your standards and achieve more in life, be more happy and joyful, then quit as I did.

You will feel and see the difference. Remember it's not just coffee that's the poison. It's the caffeine that is in the coffee. The same kind of false high can be found in all of those energy drinks, highly caffeinated colas, and many more beverages. Cut them out of your day and see how your life can improve. There are plenty of other ways to gain energy. You don't have to drink your energy.

Understanding Dopamine Opens Up Your Awareness of Happiness

Dopamine has been given a bad reputation over the years. This is because it is commonly associated with all the bad behaviors you can do, such as lust, sex, and adultery.

When we talk about removing toxins from the body, it's important to look at dopamine. It is a chemical produced by the brain and is what helps to keep us functioning. However, too much of a good thing can be very dangerous.

Did You Know This?

Virtually every drug will increase dopamine transmission. This includes the illegal ones like morphine and cocaine, as well as the OTC ones like nicotine and amphetamine.

When there are more dopamine neurotransmissions, there are longer periods of reward, which is what makes them dangerous. There's a greater risk of abusing the drugs when these reward periods are experienced, which explains why many people develop addictions to these various drugs.

What Dopamine Does In The Body

Dopamine is responsible for influencing a variety of functions within the human body, including motor function (how the muscles work), motivation, and pleasure.

When we talk about being happy and doing things that put us in a better mood, it seems contradictory to think that you could have something that gives you a sense of rewards yet is not particularly good for us.

However, what is really happening is that it's the abuse of a substance or drug that causes super high levels of dopamine that is the problem, not small amounts of a substance or drug. Dopamine production beyond natural levels is the problem.

How Drugs Fry The Brain

Too much exposure to drugs can change the function of the brain. The receptors decrease in receptivity when constantly exposed to drugs. The continuous use of drugs eventually dulls the receptors so that you are incapable of feeling motivated, feeling pleasure, and even having the desired motor skills. You go through life numb, in a matter of speaking.

Since it's 'normal' to feel your feelings, your body physiology drives you to continue to increase drug use as a way of trying to feel. As a result, the addiction becomes stronger.

As you take or use these drugs, they are not only affecting dopamine production. They affect the other chemicals in your brain plus they take a toll on other parts of your body. The addiction slowly starts to kill you – all because you were trying to seek more rewards than was naturally supposed to occur.

Compare Dopamine in Humans to Animals

Dopamine has been viewed as the brain chemical that makes us human. It's a chemical not found in large amounts in primates or any other animals. The other animals have it, just not a lot of it. Dopamine allows us to plan ahead and resist impulses as needed to run our life. Because dopamine is a neurotransmitter, it will control communication within the brain and determine if neurons should fire inside the brain or not.

We as Homo sapiens creatures have evolved to have more dopamine levels than other animals. Some of this has to do with what we do and what we eat. As one theory goes, it's because we are bipedals that has changed us – standing on two feet has forced some chemicals to different areas of the brain. We also eat more meat and fish, which gives us more of the precursors for dopamine.

Dopamine has been associated with impulse control, aggression, and competitiveness. We can say that these are all natural human traits, but too much of them can lead to all sorts of problems. We don't want to have too many problems with aggression, impulse control, or too much of any other feeling because it makes us hard to get along with in society. We could begin alienating those around us – and that leads to issues with overall happiness and the ability to have our needs met.

Surprise: What You Eat Creates Neurotransmitters

Neurotransmitters are produced naturally in the brain, but what we put into our body is what controls how much of the neurotransmitters the brain makes. The proteins we eat may contain L-tyrosine, the precursor amino acid for making dopamine.

The more foods we eat with this amino acid, the more dopamine is created. Since dopamine is a natural chemical the body makes, it can still be regulated. By eating more foods with tyrosine, we are simply adding fuel to the machinery.

Too Much Dopamine Versus Too Little

It is when we damage the receptors with drugs and increase the natural dopamine production through the introduction of other chemicals that we risk damaging the machine. During early development, introducing other chemicals that increase dopamine production to high levels can cause mental retardation.

This means that if you are pregnant and using these drugs, you could be affecting the dopamine levels of your unborn child; the lack of dopamine within the brain of the fetus could result in mental retardation at birth.

Various health problems are caused by dopamine problems, too. The list includes binge eating, food addictions, gambling, Alzheimer Disease, Parkinson's syndrome, schizophrenia, depression, bipolar disorders, and others.

Too much dopamine in the wrong part of the brain may also result in psychosis. If you take illegal drugs, a significant amount of dopamine is forced into the brain without the neurotransmitter receptors' ability to determine whether or not they should fire. This is why the high levels of dopamine are associated with such behaviors as euphoria, aggression, and sexual feelings.

Search out the side effects of different illegal drugs and you'll find that each has its own list of symptoms. Many of these symptoms include euphoria and aggression because of the dopamine levels. This is why people associate dopamine with the word 'bad' – they assume it is all because of illegal drugs.

What you need to be aware of is that the brain is continually producing neurotransmitters. You need dopamine in your brain to function like a normal human being. Without it, you could have problems with motor skills and the inability to plan. Too much dopamine, however, is where you run into other problems. This means you must establish a happy medium so you have just the right amount.

If you are currently noticing that you have problems with aggression, inappropriate sexual behavior, or anything else, you may want to consider the influence of dopamine levels on your physiology. High levels and low levels are just as dangerous because both will result in weakness in your body.

Dopamine Deficiency is Diagnosable

Some symptoms of a deficiency in dopamine include rapid weight gain, trouble focusing, low libido, oversleeping, and restless legs syndrome. The messages that are supposed to be sent to the brain to control muscle movement are not always reaching their destination when there's a deficiency.

Talk to your doctor about dopamine testing if you believe you have a deficiency (resulting in chronic fatigue, chronic boredom) or have too much (aggression, high libido).

A simple urine test gives a doctor the clues he needs to know to diagnose you. An imbalance can often be treated quickly enough so you can overcome any issues and begin leading a normal life once again. Prescribed supplements will bring the balance back.

Be cognizant of what's happening with your body at all times. If you notice you are exhibiting any symptoms of too much or not enough dopamine, then act. Stay away from illegal drugs. It's also a good idea to look at what you eat on a regular basis so you can fuel your dopamine levels with more of the L-tyrosine amino acid.

The only one who can control your body and keep it healthy is you. If something isn't right, you have the power to change it through the foods you eat and by seeking help from a doctor.

Making Small Changes in Diet to Affect Your Dopamine Levels

Making some small changes in the way you eat can have a dramatic effect on your mood and thus your overall emotional state. The key is not just about avoiding certain foods, however.

A big part of the key is about WHEN you feed your body because everything you eat is interconnected with your blood sugar, your brain, and your hormones. Thus, the chemicals your brain produces depend on the fine tuning of all these – and that in turn determines whether you are happy or not.

Are you eating as regularly as you should? Just about everyone gets tired and cranky when they skip a meal, so be sure that you don't. You can't drive around town without gas in your car and you can't stay happy without fuel in your body, either.

Make a conscious effort to eat throughout the day. More and more research has shown there's more to the picture than eating three meals a day. Breakfast is important and so is lunch and dinner. But those three meals are only half of it. You also need a few snacks throughout the day.

The better breakdown of food during the day for happy hormones is:

1. Breakfast

2. Mid-morning snack

3. Lunch

4. Mid-afternoon snack

5. Dinner

6. Dessert/snack

Six smaller meals keep calories and nutrients coming into your body more regularly so you have fuel. This also ensures that you don't have any tired and cranky episodes, which result from not having any food in your system. If you feel yourself getting cranky, it's likely that your blood sugar is sinking. Keep some fuel in your desk at work. Candy bars and donuts don't have a place here – you have to fuel your body with the right foods, and that is covered in the next chapter.

Eat to Avoid Mood Swings

Having more energy is always a good thing because it will allow you to do more things. Additionally, you want to eliminate mood swings whenever possible. What you put into your body (or don't put in) is going to determine whether you have a mood swing.

This is because the food used as fuel has a way of affecting your body in various ways. It's easy to blame a mood swing on a hormonal imbalance, but when you look at what causes the hormonal imbalance; it can often be traced back to diet. This is why doctors who try to help you overcome illnesses will always focus on nutrition.

The purpose of drinking should be to replenish your fluids, but what you drink may not contribute to replenishing your fluids. Water, tea, and other beverages will replenish your fluids easily. Other foods will give you the feeling that you are replenishing your fluids but are also doing other things to your body.

For example, if you down a liter of regular soda, you are also feeding your body a significant amount of sugar. You might have eliminated the thirsty feeling you had, but your body is likely on a sugar high, followed by a significant drop in energy, which will make you feel anything but happy and productive.

Use Foods To Produce Stable Emotions

When you start to eat better foods and eat them during the best times of the day, you will be a healthier person with a firmer grasp on your emotions. You can improve your happiness when you can maintain the right emotions throughout the day.

People won't be afraid to approach you and this can make all the difference in the world in terms of how you interact with people and how you generally feel throughout the day, the week, and through life.

The foods you eat and the beverages you drink can be poisons to your body as well as to your emotional well being. Watch how your body responds to certain foods. Becoming more aware of your eating habits and how you feel after eating certain foods can tell you a lot about what you should and shouldn't be eating.

Timing of Foods is Critical to Your Neurotransmitter Production

If you don't feel good about yourself or don't feel good physically after eating a particular food, then you probably shouldn't eat it anymore. The types of foods are important but what also is important is when you eat them.

Foods may not be poisons when you eat them at the right times of the day. Get into the habit of reading labels, eating fresh foods, and eating six smaller meals. Feed your body the good foods, not the bad foods and watch how your mood and your overall ability to be happy changes when you remove the poisons from your diet on a daily basis.

When you do this, you will feel a positive change throughout your entire body. You are going to have more energy, have fewer mood swings, and be in a better mood all the time. This doesn't mean that you will eliminate unhappiness from your life.

However, when you have a better fuel coursing through your body, little things don't bother you as much. You can overlook small obstacles and focus on the bigger things – and this can eliminate a significant amount of stress. This means that removing the poisons also removes some of the stress and negativity currently in your life.

Additionally, you will have more energy to deal with obstacles that stand in your way and have a more positive outlook in life that will propel you forward to reach your no matter what is going on. Removing the toxins will help, but you also have to know what you should be putting into your body.

Exercise 7. What's Your Why?

1. Write a small paragraph about why you want to have more energy, vitality, be more productive and sleep better.

2. If you regularly eat too many poisons mentioned in this chapter, write another paragraph about the consequences of this on your health, the quality of your life, and your relationships if you don't change your lifestyle.

3. Take Action. I know you are an achiever, and if you have read this book up to this point, you want more in your life. So why wait to make a shift in your life? Decide today which foods you are no longer eating or drinking from today on, or at least reduce their intake. Make a commitment and tell your partner/ friend about your new lifestyle.

Chapter 7
Eat Better Foods

"You must take personal responsibility. You cannot change the circumstances, the seasons, or the wind, but you can change yourself. That is something you have charge of."

— im Rohn

If you have to remove the poisons, an empty hole arises in your life. What should you be eating? There is no exact formula for what you should be eating, but your doctor and nutritionist may likely make some recommendations.

The bottom line is eating more fresh fruits and vegetables and drinking a lot more water. Health benefits transfer to you from the phytonutrients found in leafy vegetables.

You have to provide the right foods for your body. If you don't do it, who will? When you don't eat the right foods, toxins enter into your body; the very thing you don't want. This means to focus on various foods and their health benefits. Pick and choose what your body needs based upon how it is performing right now.

Water is a great beverage that offers an array of health benefits. It's calorie-free, so you can stay hydrated without consuming any empty calories in the process. When you drink enough water, it can promote weight loss, boost your immune system, and flush out toxins.

Water relieves fatigue and increases your available energy, which only makes sense when you consider 70% of your body and 90% of your brain is comprised of water. Water could be your natural remedy for headaches, cramps, and even constipation.

What you put into your body is an important factor in how your body performs and even the amount of energy you have, your temperament, and overall personality. Remove the poisons, add in some healthier foods and watch how you become happier in your life.

Green Tea vs. Coffee

There are over 180 million people in the U.S. alone that rely on coffee to make it through the day. The caffeine is buzzing through the body and gets you through the morning and every other part in the day where you seem to just drag.

If you're a coffee drinker, you're not alone. However, you need to know what it's doing to your body so that you can have a moment of clarity before you brew your next cup.

Coffee is rarely organic, which means it is being treated by a lot of pesticides that could result in all sorts of health problems. Long-term use of coffee may also result in higher cholesterol levels in the blood and a higher risk of heart disease as well as osteoporosis. This means that the beverage you drink every morning could be putting you at risk of becoming sick.

Have you ever drunk coffee on an empty stomach? If so, you know that your stomach may get upset with coffee.

The reason is because your stomach produces hydrochloric acid when it senses coffee. Your stomach should only be producing hydrochloric acid to digest solid foods.

This means that the acid will stay in your stomach, resulting in more gas, and potentially even health problems like colon cancer. It can also lead to ulcers due to the high level of acidity.

Coffee may also prevent your body from absorbing iron – and affect the way you absorb all other vitamins and minerals from foods you eat, even if you take supplements. This means you may be depriving your body of the calcium, magnesium, zinc, and other minerals it needs.

Have you ever noticed irritability after drinking coffee? It's the caffeine. Coffee can turn on the stress hormones in your body and make it difficult to relax. As a result, your body is in a jittery and tense state, not a state you want to be in for very long.

You may want to drink another cup to help ease the tension, but it's what you're drinking that's causing the problem. This is exactly how you end up with an addiction. When I first realized this, I was completely stunned. I used to drink coffee for this exact reason… to relax, but it was making me more anxious and irritable.

Today, I drink green tea or black tea with squeezed lemon in it, and afterwards am energized and relaxed. Quitting coffee is a very important step if you want to achieve better health. Of course, also reduce alcohol and smoking. Smoking does not have its own chapter in this book because we all have been drilled on what smoking does to our body.

What can you do about a coffee addiction? Give up your cup of coffee in the morning – and throughout the rest of the day. If you must have it, go for organic and make sure you're not drinking it on an empty stomach. Even better, and drink green tea.

If you're worried about disturbing your daily routine of going to the coffee shop every morning on your way to work, rest assured that the average coffee shop has green tea on the menu – and you can get it hot or cold just as you can get coffee.

What are the health benefits of tea? Tea can assist in hydrating the body and even reduce the risk of developing various tumors and cancers. Tea also has the ability to keep you going for longer time periods during the day. The rush of caffeine in tea boosts your energy levels, but it doesn't have the short stay that coffee does.

Green tea is filled with antioxidants called catechins. These catechins allow you to maintain a fresh and vibrant feeling for a lot longer. Catechins and other medicinal constituents in tea have been proven to reduce free radicals roaming around in your body so you can literally improve your health with every sip that you take. Green tea has also been shown to speed up metabolism, which is why many people are now drinking it or taking it in capsules as a way to help lose weight.

While coffee has been shown to promote osteoporosis, green tea can help to reduce the risks. This means that by drinking more tea, you can reduce the risks of what you may have done by drinking coffee every day for how-ever many years straight.

Tea can also boost your immune system, so it's important to promote this system however you can. The next time you're sick, you may find that your body pushes past the infection a lot faster so there is nothing for you to worry about. It can also maintain whiter teeth, as coffee is often associated with the yellowing of teeth.

When it comes to drinking something in the morning or any other time of the day, tea is the better choice over coffee. It can improve the health of your body and won't give you the jittery, tense feeling that coffee does. Overall, it's going to give you the boost of energy that you need without playing with your mood or emotions. This allows you to keep your emotions in check easier throughout the day because you don't have a substance altering anything without your knowledge.

A simple switch of what you drink in the morning can provide you with the ability to be happier and healthier. You can maintain a smile for longer throughout the day because something going into your body isn't going to stress you out for no apparent reason.

There are plenty of things that you can do to help eliminate toxins and generally improve the way that you eat so that you can improve the way that you feel. It's simple to do, especially when you know the 'why' behind why certain foods make you feel the way that they do.

10 Foods to a Happier Outlook

What you eat can affect your mood. This has nothing to do with being an emotional eater, though your cravings can tell you a lot about the foods that you are deficient in. That is something that will be covered in a moment.

The brain is what ultimately controls mood and that means that you need to have a healthy cognitive system. Some nutrients have a deeper impact on brain function than others.

Various foods that contain B6, B12, calcium, folate, chromium, magnesium, iron, and omega-3 fatty acids along with zinc can boost your mood and combat depression at the same time. This means you want to eat foods that contain high levels of these nutrients, and there are 10 listed below:

1. Collard Greens

Your body needs calcium to be happy and that's because it may reduce depression – especially PMS-related depression. Collard greens are packed with calcium, so it's a good idea to load up on this veggie. You need 1000 mg of calcium a day and if you don't want collard greens, you can also turn to ricotta, milk, kale, and low-fat yogurt.

2. Mashed Potatoes

Mashed potatoes are high in chromium, and so are grape juice, broccoli, and turkey breasts. Chromium is a good thing to have great levels of from your diet because it regulates insulin and positively affects your mood. Have you noticed you are moody when you're hungry? It may have to do with a low blood sugar issue and chromium can help. 25 mcg for women and 35 mcg for men are recommended on a daily basis.

3. Avocado

Avocados are full of nutrients including folate, which supports serotonin (the happy chemical in your brain), as well as helps the brain manage many different functions. Boosting folate levels could help in many ways, including solving a chapped lips problem. Folate is found in Brussels sprouts and asparagus. You want to get the daily requirement of 400 mcg of folate in a day; more if you are deficient.

4. Beef Rib Eye

You have permission to eat a beef rib eye on a regular basis and that's because it delivers high levels of iron. Iron oxygenates your blood, which in turn energizes you and aids in the strength of your muscles. Low levels could cause fatigue and depression. You need iron daily, and it can be provided from soybeans, lentils, and dark turkey meat. The recommended daily amounts are 18 mg for menstruating women and 8 mg for men.

5. Almonds

Almonds are a great snack. Because they are packed with magnesium, they give you the boost that your body needs to avoid stress, irritability, and fatigue – all which can have a negative impact on your mood. Almonds help you create serotonin, which is the happiness chemical in your brain. If you don't want to eat almonds, there's always edamame, cashews, and spinach that are high in magnesium as a substitute. Strive for 310 mg a day of magnesium daily if you're a woman, or 400 mg magnesium if you're a man.

6. Salmon

Salmon is high in omega-3 fatty acids, a nutrient needed to reduce fatigue, depression, memory decline, and even mood swings. More and more research confirms that omega-3 fasts are important for brain health, and salmon is a good choice to get it. Other sources include chia seeds, spinach, or even Atlantic herring.

7. Chickpeas

Chickpeas, the main ingredient in hummus, are high in B6. This vitamin contributes to the process whereby neurotransmitters send messages to the brain. A deficiency of vitamin B6 could result in confusion as well as depression. Yellow fin tuna and chicken breasts are good sources of vitamin B6. The recommended daily amount is only 1.3 mg.

8. Cheese

Mozzarella cheese and tuna are high in vitamin B12. If you have low levels of this vitamin, you can experience fatigue and even slow reasoning ability and decision-making. Who wants these symptoms? Don't take a chance. The recommended daily intake is 2.4 mcg per day.

9. Eggs

Eggs are a source of Vitamin D, which protects your bone density and is also responsible for regulating moods. Without enough sun exposure, you'll develop a deficiency, and doctors estimate that more than half of the population is low in this important vitamin.

Increasing your intake of this vitamin through food and supplements is critical to staying in a good mood – and preventing diabetes. Chandelle mushrooms, milk, and swordfish are good sources to help keep levels high but you need to determine how high your levels are right now. The recommended daily intake used to be around 600 IU but many health experts say that 2000 IU per day is better when levels have already hit the level not associated with deficiency.

10. Cashews

Cashews are one of the foods that are very high in zinc and can help support your immune system and reduce depression. If you find you are suddenly depressed, it is possible you do not have enough zinc in your body. If you don't want to eat cashews, you can also opt for pork loin, Swiss cheese, or roasted pumpkin seeds. Men need about 11 mg per day and women need about 8 mg per day.

With so many different foods, you can truly enjoy good meals and feel happy afterward. There is no rule that says you have to eat all these foods all the time. However, if you can find recipes that incorporate one or two of them into your diet on a daily basis, it can help you be healthier and happier.

There may be other foods not on this list that you find will consistently bring you happiness. Don't exclude them because they're not included here. Everyone is unique and you may have some foods that you love and make you happy; don't ignore the input your body gives you about foods.

Have You Tried Smoothies Yet?

Have you discovered the benefits of a green smoothie? These beverages pack in so many vitamins and nutrients into one glass that they make a nutritionist smile.

A smoothie is capable of feeding your body all that it needs in a 4-hour period of time and will boost your energy level. More food companies are offering green smoothies though you can easily shop for ingredients such as kale, spinach, avocado, berries, parsley, cilantro, lemon, citrus fruits, yogurt, bee pollen, nutritional yeast, lecithin, chia seeds, flax seeds, almonds, walnuts, and pecans, and make your own. Smoothies are easy to master and taste delicious.

Whether you choose foods from this list or use your own list, it's important to identify the difference between foods that make you happy and foods you are craving.

Food cravings may be mental and emotional more than physical. Some cravings should not be fed because they will bring you unhappiness later on – and this is when you need to exercise self-control.

Food Cravings Mean Pay Attention to Your Body

Now, here's a little more about food cravings. When you eat healthy meals, you fuel your body with what it needs and that makes you feel good about yourself. A lot of your cravings need to be interpreted properly so your body receives the best fuel possible. What this means is you have to think about why you are craving foods in the first place.

If you're craving chocolate, it may be your body's cry for magnesium. This means you should reach for nuts and seeds instead.

If you're craving fatty foods, your body may be crying for calcium. Instead, reach for cheese and leafy green vegetables.

While chocolate and potato chips might make you feel good initially, you'll quickly notice that the short-term happiness fades fast, especially if you gain weight. This means learn to be cautious about the foods you eat.

The 10 foods in this chapter are given as suggestions to help you maintain the levels of nutrients your body needs to combat depression, raise energy levels, and make sure your brain is making plenty of serotonin. When your brain functions at its best, you will be in a better mood – and that leads to a whole lot of happiness to share with the world at large.

You can always meet with a nutritionist to find out what your body needs. If you need more vitamins and minerals to help your body function well, you still need a little direction as to what to take. Don't guess at this. Supplements you choose on your own are all well and good, but the best source of vitamins and minerals are the foods you eat on a regular basis. Foods are absorbed at maximum absorption levels while supplements are not.

Start eating the right food and watch how much more energy you have during the day. Your body will be at peak level, which means it's not burning more energy than necessary digesting and excreting the toxins or doing anything else. You will have more energy, a better memory, and an overall better state of health once the right food goes in – and that means you are on your way to being happier because you are healthier.

The Dopamine Diet

Too many of the drugs that lower dopamine production can cause you to overeat as a way of giving your body more of the feel good feeling. You may be eating and overeating as a way of compensating for the low dopamine production.

This is because your food and sugar cravings are kicking in to compensate so you will eat more in an attempt to get those nutrients you need even though you're not hungry. This can lead to weight gain and overall depression.

Higher levels of dopamine can reduce your binge eating, so eat foods high in tyrosine. Why Tyrosine? It is the amino acid building block responsible for dopamine production. As you eat foods rich in L-tyrosine, the brain receptors for dopamine will actually reactivate. You can increase your pleasure levels through smaller amounts of food.

There are some foods high in L-tyrosine you may want to incorporate into your diet. Some of them include:

- Chicken

- Duck

- Wheat germ

- Fava beans

- Oatmeal

- Mustard greens

- Edamame

- Ricotta cheese

- Dark chocolate

The best thing you can do is incorporate one of these foods into each meal throughout the day.

Sample Recipes

Where can you find recipes? They are everywhere online. Below are four recipes that incorporate four foods from the list. As you learn new recipes, make sure you take them one step further by incorporating the recipe into your regular diet.

This way you will improve your dopamine levels in a natural way. This ensures you don't have to overeat and you can get the happy feelings your body needs without having to turn to any illegal drugs. It's the healthiest way to act and plus, the foods are delicious!

Wheat Germ Oven-Fried Chicken

Prep time: 15 minutes Bake time: 45 minutes Servings: 8

Ingredients:

2 Tablespoons olive oil
½ teaspoon salt
½ teaspoon pepper
½ teaspoon paprika
¼ teaspoon cayenne pepper
½ cup low-fat buttermilk
¾ cup toasted wheat germ
2 eggs, beaten
4 cups crushed corn flakes
4 large chicken legs, 4 chicken thighs (skin removed)

Instructions:

1. Preheat oven to 350 degrees.

2. Use a baking sheet with sides and oil it.

3. Mix seasonings and wheat germ in a bowl. Then place buttermilk, eggs, and corn flakes each in their own bowls.

4. Take chicken, one piece at a time, and dip into buttermilk bowl, then wheat germ mix bowl, then egg bowl, and then the corn flakes. Place on the baking sheet.

5. Bake in oven until golden and crisp, approximately 45 minutes. Serve.

Lemon Garlic Fava Beans with Mushrooms

Prep time: 10 minutes Cook time: 30 minutes Servings: 4

Ingredients:

2 teaspoons olive oil
1 red onion, cut into thin half moons
3 cloves garlic, minced
1 Tablespoon chopped thyme, fresh
8 oz. cremini mushrooms, sliced in half
2 Tablespoons breadcrumbs, plain
2 cups vegetable broth
½ teaspoon salt
Zest and juice from ½ lemon
Fresh black pepper
3 cups cooked fava beans

Instructions:

1. Preheat a pan on stove at medium heat.

2. Sauté onion with oil and salt for 5 to 7 minutes, or until lightly golden.

3. Add garlic and thyme and continue to sauté for 1 minute. Add mushrooms and sauté, about 5 minutes.

4. Add breadcrumbs and toss to coat, cooking on medium high heat. Crumbs should be toasted in 3 to 5 minutes.

5. Add broth, salt and pepper, juice, zest, and beans. Bring to a boil. Let reduce and thicken, approximately 7 minutes.

Noodles with Duck Breast, Dried Cherries, and Edamame

Prep time: 10 minutes Cook time: 15 minutes Servings: 4

Ingredients:

8 oz. wide egg noodles
3 lbs. boneless duck breast, thawed and skinned
2 teaspoons salt
1 teaspoon pepper
4 Tablespoons olive oil
2 cups dried sweet cherries
4 cups frozen shelled edamame
2 cups dry white wine
2 cups chicken broth (low sodium)
2 teaspoons chopped rosemary, fresh
8 Tablespoons unsalted butter

Instructions:

1. Cook noodles according to package. Add edamame when there are three minutes remaining on noodles cooking time. Continue cooking, then drain.

2. Cube duck into ½ inch pieces. Toss with half of the salt and half of the pepper.

3. Heat a nonstick pan at medium high heat with olive oil and add duck. Cook for about 3 minutes on each side or until brown.

4. Add cherries and cook one minute. Then transfer duck and cherries to a bowl.

5. Add wine, broth, and rosemary along with remaining salt and pepper to the skillet. Bring to a boil and scrape sides to get brown bits into liquid.

6. When liquid is reduced by half (in approximately 4 minutes), stir in the butter and then toss with the noodles and duck. Serve immediately.

Dark Chocolate Ricotta Mousse

Prep time: 5 minutes Servings: 4

Ingredients:

3 oz. dark chocolate
1 lb. ricotta cheese
1-½ teaspoons vanilla extract
1 Tablespoon honey

Instructions:

1. Melt chocolate squares in a double boiler. Stir until it is completely melted.

2. Then combine the melted chocolate, vanilla, honey, and ricotta into a food processor. Process until smooth and creamy, approximately 30 seconds.

3. Pour into a baking pan.

4. Refrigerate for about an hour and serve.

Tyrosine Helps Stop Food Cravings

In addition to eating these different foods, you will also want to consider taking an L-tyrosine supplement. This is something that can be taken twice a day – once in the morning and then another one between lunch and dinner. The normal dosage is between 500 and 1,000 mg. It is a stimulating supplement; so don't take it on an empty stomach or right before bed.

To avoid any health issues, it's always advisable to talk to your doctor about taking any supplement before you actually go on it. Some blood testing may be required before you get the seal of approval from your doctor. If you have a history of hypertension or an abnormal heartbeat, you may be advised against taking the supplement; then you will want to focus on diet changes alone.

After taking the supplement for approximately four to six weeks, it will have reached a sufficient level of effectiveness and cravings will be reduced. You won't be overeating and your sweet cravings have diminished greatly.

Will you benefit from this diet?

Yes, you will if you:

- Have late night snack cravings.

- Eat even when full.

- Become tired or irritable when you eat fewer of your favorite foods

The Dopamine Diet has been discussed in detail in the medical field via medical journals because of its ability to control hunger cravings and create weight loss quickly and effectively. Your body may be telling you that it needs food that it really doesn't because your neurotransmitters are not in line. Unhealthy spikes of food cravings need to be controlled and the diet has been proven to work.

Dr. Oz has suggested that you have breakfast, lunch, and dinner with ingredients high in L-tyrosine and even add in a dessert from time to time.

As long as you eat foods high in L-tyrosine throughout the day on a daily basis, you are doing something good for the body. You can naturally suppress food cravings and be healthier for this simple change. While you don't have to eat all foods on the list in this chapter, it is advantageous to eat as many of them for variety. Two or three of these foods daily can make a significant transformation.

Once your dopamine levels are raised in a healthy way, you will find you are more motivated, more passionate, and generally in a happier, healthier state of mind.

Exercise 8. Tweaking Your Diet To Include Healthy Foods

1. Make a weekly menu plan, and include some of the healthy foods mentioned above.

2. Then create a grocery list of the foods in your healthy diet. A healthy lifestyle starts by making the right decisions at the health food or grocery store.

3. Start recording what you eat on a daily basis. This is easily done via today's technology. I use this app to record my eating: http://www.myfitnesspal.com/mobile/iphone The app is free and a powerful tool to help you stay on a healthy diet.

Chapter 8
Explore the Benefits of Meditation

"Happiness is not something ready made. It comes from your own actions."

— Dalai Lama

How Do You See Meditation?

You may currently see meditation as a form of sitting quietly and reflecting. This is not entirely accurate. It is not only deep concentration and it doesn't involve exercising or a loss of control.

Instead, meditation is a form of transformation. In meditation, you visualize what is going on and what you want to have happen within the deeper areas of your mind. There are a variety of techniques that can encourage clarity, concentration, as well as emotional positivity. Depending upon the practice that you choose, it will be very easy for you to reach a positive state of meditation.

When you start to prepare for meditation, first make sure your environment is calming. There should not be a lot of background noise and you want to be alone. If you have any kind of anxiety, fear, personal sorrows, or anything else preventing you from becoming happy, you can meditate your way through these in order to reach a deeper understanding that there are some things out of your control.

Meditation may be something you have tried in the past. Whether you have tried and succeeded or tried and failed, it should be a part of your everyday life.

Even 20 minutes worth of meditation can be life-changing and allow you to relax so you don't allow stress to overcome your life. As you have read throughout this book, stress is one of the worst things for you, your brain, and your body. When you can learn to eliminate it, you experience more positive thoughts, have more positive things to say to those around you, and reach higher levels of happiness.

It is hard to smile and reach a true level of happiness when you are constantly stressed out. Your mind is going in 1 million directions and you say what is on your mind before thinking about how it may affect others.

This means you are not happy and everyone around you will not be happy either. You don't want to be the symbol of doom and gloom within your circle of friends; prevent this from happening simply by exploring meditation in a more thorough way. You will learn the health benefits, the way that affects the brain, and effective ways to meditate on a daily basis.

What Happens to the Brain

Various things take place within your brain when you meditate; modern science has shown significant differences. When the brain is meditating. Information is not processed as actively as it would on a normal basis.

Beta waves, which provide an overall calming effect, are decreased. If you feel as though your mind is going in 1 million directions on a regular basis, this is because your brain is processing so much information. Within a 20-minute meditation session, you can eliminate a significant amount of this processing in order to relieve stress.

Things are always happening 24/7 within every aspect of your brain.

The frontal lobe is responsible for planning functions, reasoning, and emotions. When you are meditating, the frontal cortex of this lobe is turned off and you do not have any self-conscious awareness.

The parietal lobe is responsible for processing sensory information and orienting you into space and time. During meditation, this type of brain activity is dramatically slowed because you are not aware of time and space. If you have reached a deep level of meditation, you have transcended the concepts of time and space completely.

The thalamus part of your brain is the part that focuses your attention and helps organize sensory data. The flow of incoming information is reduced dramatically during meditation simply because you are not aware of what is going on. The flow of information can be considered a trickle during meditation.

Finally, there is the reticular formation, which receives all incoming stimuli and alerts the brain to what is going on. The signal is dramatically reduced during meditation, which means you are less likely to get aroused when you are in a meditative state.

Everything that goes on inside of your brain affects your health. Meditation is responsible for focusing attention and becoming aware of when attention drifts. This can benefit you in many ways, because your focus improves even when you are not meditating. It has been proven that meditation provides a lasting effect, which means that even when you have gone back to your normal activities, you will still have a sharper level of focus.

Any time you can improve the overall function of your brain, it is going to be beneficial. Sometimes just slowing down your brain will allow it to work better. When busy and stressed, your mind is spinning at a rate that is unhealthy. Meditating can help slow it down in all regards. If you could look at an image of your brain on a normal day while working and thinking, and then compare this to an image of your brain when you were meditating, you would see the differences – and want to meditate more often. These positive differences help keep you healthy and sane – and allow you to achieve more happiness in your life.

Benefits of Meditation

There are countless benefits to meditation. You can decide how many times you want to meditate in a week, but it is recommended that you do so with regularity and frequency to experience all the health benefits and reach a higher level of happiness that is sustainable. When you have an external stimuli affecting your ability to be happy, maintaining a laser sharp focus on what you can and cannot control is important – and meditation can provide this focus.

Increased immunity is one of the many health benefits from meditation. As you relax, the functioning of the immune system improves. What would it be like for you to experience a greater resistance to viruses, tumors, and infections?

Worldwide studies prove how meditation can help cancer patients. The strong level of muscular relaxation that takes place during meditation can also assist with chronic pain.

Emotional Balance and Increased Fertility

Emotional balance is also gained during meditation. Throughout your life, you may have had a tortured and traumatized ego. You may also experience neurotic behavior from time to time. When you establish an emotional balance, you are free from your ego as well as any kind of behaviors that are unhealthy.

You will have the ability to cleanse your consciousness of any memories that repeat themselves. Meditation allows you to eliminate some of the burdens you carry on a daily basis, so you stop feeling weighed down by them.

Studies have shown that fertility is increased as a result of deep relaxation. Especially in today's times, many people walk around feeling so stressed. As you learn to relax, you can take your level of fertility higher. It can help men and women alike, which means you have the ability to boost both male and female fertility.

Improved Digestive Functions and Less Stress

Irritable bowel syndrome, otherwise known as IBS, can be relieved as a result of deep relaxation and meditation as well. Patients with irritable bowel syndrome who have practiced meditation have noticed they can lessen symptoms of diarrhea, bloating, and constipation dramatically. Research has been done at the University of New York, as well as various other universities to prove this.

When there is a lot of stress in your life, it can lead to inflammation in the body. This makes you more susceptible to develop arthritis, heart disease, psoriasis, other skin conditions, asthma, and other health problems.

When you take the time to relax and meditate, you can prevent and treat your own symptoms. This is because relaxation and meditation switches the stress response off. Meditation has even been used clinically in order to improve various symptoms.

If you compare someone who does and does not meditate, you will notice a difference in how they handle stressful situations. This is because the mind has learned to filter various events and emotions. While upsetting thoughts can occur in either person, the person who meditates will be able to see the upsetting thought as just another thought and let it go while the other person is going to allow it to blossom into a level of rage.

You can experience a number of these benefits on your own through meditation. You can lower blood pressure, reduce inflammation, and give your immune system a boost. You deserve to reach happiness and this can be done in a variety of ways.

Meditation is not something you can learn overnight because it needs practice, but through various techniques, you can reach the meditative state that helps heal the mind and focus thoughts so that they do not overwhelm you.

Effective Ways to Meditate

If you want to reach the higher levels of concentration that have been discussed, it is important that you learn how to meditate effectively. There are several different types of meditation. Strive to understand the best possible posture for it, which ones are the transforming meditations, and which ones use breathing meditation techniques. This will help you reach a higher level of transcendence faster so you can relieve stress and begin to reach the happiness you are choosing in life.

Breathing meditations are of the utmost importance because these calm your mind and help you develop some level of inner peace. Breathing meditations may be used alone or in conjunction with other meditation techniques. Choose a quiet place to sit and meditate.

The best posture is cross-legged on the floor, though you can use a chair as well – as long as there is not a lot of stimuli in the chair – such as a ripped seat cushion or a massaging mode turned on. Close your eyes; breathe through your nostrils and out your mouth. You want to take long and deep breaths and feel distress, leaving each time you exhale.

Distractions are Handled

The first few times you inhale, your mind will be busy with everything that is happening. The idea is to close your mind to what is going on. Ignore any of the external stimuli and focus on your breathing. The only thing that should concern you right now is breathing in through your nostrils and out through your mouth. You can do this as many times as needed so your mind settles on the breath alone.

At some point, all the distracting thoughts will leave your mind. You will be left with a sense of relaxation and a sense of inner peace. At this point, you have reached the preliminary stage of meditation and can then move on to an additional stage where you begin to focus your energy on a particular concept.

This may be a particular problem or emotion you are dealing with and one that is important to identify to bring about solutions. Understanding the best way to deal with your problem and how to eliminate your emotional bond to it will be part of the solution. Identifying emotions surrounding the problem ensures that these emotions do not follow you around on a daily basis, influence other decisions and actions, and weigh you down.

Consider Using CDs to Help You Meditate

Many people find it beneficial to use music or even meditational CDs to help you relax. There are some great CDs on the market that will talk you through the state of meditation. They utilize a soft, soothing voice that will describe what you need to do through each of the stages.

It will take the time to walk you through everything so you know what needs to be done. After you have reached the level desired, the CD will turn to music, allowing you to focus on what is going on inside of your mind as opposed to listening to the words on the CD.

I used to be stressed all the time, worrying about everything, business, how I looked, and went throughout my day making my family and business partners happy. One day I decided to become more spiritual and began meditating on a regular base.

I bought an online meditation program (https://chopracentermeditation. com/experience), and my life shifted to a better quality of life, more balanced, more peaceful ideas, and more hope for my future. I completely recommend meditation to become more spiritual in your life. By starting to do something for your mind or spirit, you can gain a better quality of life, become happier and achieve peace of mind.

You can combine meditation with yoga as a way to gain more clarity, more positive benefits for the body, and even various postures to assist with meditation. Learning how to flex your body can help with the flow of energy, otherwise known as chi. As you begin to improve the flow of energy, you can experience more health benefits and thus achieve happiness through another avenue.

Exercise 9. Start Meditating

1. While meditating, think and imagine five things you are grateful for in your life. By focusing on what you have (it could be your health, beautiful children, lovely wife, or just that you are alive), you will feel a sense of internal wealth, peace and happiness).

2. Meditate for at least five minutes.

3. Do your meditation as often as you can, every day or at least a couple times a week.

Chapter 9
Yoga and How it Helps the Body

"Sleep is the best meditation."

— Dalai Lama

The definition of yoga varies depending on the person. It has been practiced for thousands of years and originated in India. It is a way of creating harmony between the mind, body, and spirit. This union is achieved through physical manipulation of your body into and various poses, commonly known as an asana. There is also a level of meditation involved with yoga because of deep breathing techniques as well as achieving a level of calmness when you practice yoga.

Yoga brings various health benefits; many doctors have begun telling patients to use yoga as a way to strengthen their body and rehabilitate muscle strength. There are different types of yoga practices, and many of them are built on ancient philosophies. Yoga often involves stretching the body and holding poses for extended periods of time as a way of improving the flow of energy, as well as centering the mind.

Your spiritual well being could be enhanced or dramatically affected by practicing yoga. When your well being is stronger, your happiness follows. Meditation will enhance your mental and spiritual well being, but the corresponding physical activity should also be noted. It's the combination that can make you healthier and stronger – and help to release some endorphins along the way.

Types of Yoga

With all the different types of yoga, how do you know which one to start with? You might even want to practice a few types of yoga. Some types are more involved while others are more advanced. If you do not have a lot of flexibility, start off with the basics and then move into the advanced poses once you feel more comfortable. The idea is to work with your body and not to challenge it too much. If you hurt yourself while staying in a pose, you won't be happy and will have missed the entire point of this type of exercise.

Bikram Yoga: This form of yoga involves literally turning up the heat. In most instances, it is performed in 105° heat, as well as 40% humidity. There are only 26 poses – easy for beginners, but it will make you sweat. The benefit of the high heat is that you forget about all the things going on in your life because you will be focusing purely on achieving poses in the heat.

Hatha Yoga: If you have experienced problems with your joints, this form of yoga is a good choice because it will involve very gentle movements. It will allow you to wind down at night and help restore your body from stress you have experienced.

Vinyasa Yoga: This yoga can sometimes be referred to as flow because you are flowing through all of the different poses. You will always start with the sun salutation, though. After that, the classes will never be similar. This is considered one of the most popular forms of yoga.

Kundalini Yoga: If you are familiar with the flow of energy, this form of yoga is going to focus on your lower spine, an area where the root chakra is located. The poses will work out your core area and each session can be a very intense workout. Expect the release of endorphins to make you feel great afterwards.

Ashtanga Yoga: This form of yoga is commonly referred to as power yoga. It is one of the more physically demanding types of yoga and ideal for someone who is an athlete or who has the strength to push their body to the next level.

Iyengar Yoga: This form of yoga utilizes blocks, straps, harnesses, and even cushions. It relies on these various props to assist with body alignment. If you need rehabilitation of a past injury, this may be the form of yoga that is right for you.

Anusara Yoga: This form of yoga is commonly described as "heart open-ing" and involves a lot of poses such as backbends. Don't try this one on your own, as you will need an instructor to walk you through all the different poses.

Restorative Yoga: This may be the best form of yoga to decrease stress. After a long day of work or when you want to quiet your mind, restorative yoga could be your choice. It is best combined with various types of meditation.

Jivamukti Yoga: This form of yoga is relatively new and practiced in New York City, where it was emerged in 1984. Expect chanting and vinyasa flow, as well as a vegetarian diet. This form can help manage the body on many levels and provides various benefits to achieve happiness.

Prenatal Yoga: When you are pregnant and stressed out, you can still experience the benefits of yoga with this special prenatal version. In this type of yoga, there is a particular focus on breathing and can provide core work that will help you to regain your pre-baby body.

With so many different forms of yoga to choose from, you never get bored. As you learn the different poses, either by attending yoga classes in person or practicing them at home via DVDs, you can determine when and where you should do each of them.

One example of how to mix them up is this: Attend a vinyasa yoga class every week, perform bikram yoga while you're at the gym, and before you go to bed, strike up some restorative yoga poses.

When you are familiar with several forms of yoga, you can use them throughout various times in your life. Some weeks of your life will be more stressful than others and you may choose to combine yoga with meditation as a way to achieve focus once again in your life.

As life becomes more stressful, it's easy to lose focus. The best way to get your focus back is through meditation and yoga by using yoga postures that you are now more familiar with and which allow the flow of energy to course more effectively through your body.

How do you know what form of yoga is right for you? There is no easy answer to this question. The best thing to do is try several different forms and see which one makes you the happiest.

The overall goal here is to reach a higher level of happiness, so if you are doing a particular type of yoga that is hurting you or not helping you to reach happiness, it's not for you. Give yourself time to try a few different classes and gain an appreciation for the poses. Learn the right angles for your body. If you do not maintain the proper poses, you could hurt yourself and hinder the flow of energy.

By working with a yoga instructor for a short time in the beginning, you will start to understand what a proper poses looks like. This way you can achieve a higher level of balance and ensure that you are not wasting your time while practicing yoga at any time. You can practice yoga at home, at work, in the gym, or even in the park; all are socially acceptable. There is no right or wrong place to practice as long as you are in a peaceful environment.

How Yoga Can Create Happiness

Yoga offers many benefits that can improve your life. There have been studies that explain how hitting the mats could be beneficial to you.

Yoga is considered a way to make you happy. The reason for this is the asanas are designed to raise the chemicals of your brain known as GABA (Gamma-aminobutyric acid). Low levels of GABA have been linked to depression. When you increase the chemicals within your brain, you reduce your chances of developing depression – and this makes you a happier person by default.

If you are dealing with body aches and pains, it can be difficult to force a smile, let alone have a positive outlook on life. Many people report that lower back pain, and various other aches and pains can be eliminated by yoga sessions throughout the week.

Some research studies have shown that two 90-minute yoga classes every week for six months can dramatically reduce soreness and improve how a person can deal with chronic pain.

It is hard to be happy when you are constantly tired. When you are tired, everything is harder to deal with. You won't have the energy to get through the day and this leads to irritability.

Yoga and Sleep

Yoga can help you get a better night sleep because you are able to hit the off switch in your brain faster. You won't have a ton of things flowing through your mind because yoga teaches you how to relax. This means that those things you mull over in your mind will not be keeping you up at night. When you can sleep eight hours a night, you will have a more positive outlook for the next day.

It has also been said that yoga can increase your sexual desires and help you to achieve orgasm faster. This may occur because your body awareness increases and anxiety is reduced – two key things that will result in better sex between the sheets. When you have intercourse, it also increases endorphins, which means that the benefits keep on coming.

Self-Confidence Improves with Yoga

Studies on men and women who participate in yoga and aerobics together in their workout schedules reveal that it's easier to maintain a healthy weight with them. What's also noted is a higher level of self-confidence.

With greater self-confidence, you can make better decisions and be more confident about your actions in a social environment, in the office, and elsewhere. Additionally, yoga helps a bit with strength training – and this tones your body. You feel more confident in the clothes you wear, which in turn catapults you to even higher levels of confidence. Happiness is the result.

People who practice yoga on a regular basis have significantly less amounts of cytokines inside the body. Cytokine is a protein that creates mood swings and makes you feel tired. Knowing these two facts means you can actually change the physiology of your bod by practicing yoga and control the frequency of times you feel tired and moody.

If you have never tried yoga, talk to people who swear by it – and they will help affirm the benefits. Yoga improves your body and mind and can boost your self-confidence to higher levels than ever felt before. You choose the level of yoga you want to start with, and as you gain confidence with all of the different poses, move to more advanced versions.

How Often Do You Have to Practice?

You don't have to practice yoga daily. The health benefits are felt by practicing yoga approximately 2 hours a week. This can be in the form of one hour a day twice a week, or 30 minutes a day four times a week. Fit it in when your schedule allows. To make it work for you, fit it in at least a few times each week to gain all the benefits.

If you're anything like me, in your journey to ultimately achieve happiness, yoga may be one of the tools that help get you there. Truth be told, yoga doesn't have to be in the equation at all. It's not true that you cannot find happiness if yoga is not in your life or that yoga is essential to your happiness.

However, there are scientifically proven benefits about yoga. It is a low impact activity on the body and can improve your moods and your health. Whether you think it will help or not, try it for a week and see how it can lift your spirits and provide you with some added physical benefits at the same time.

Chapter 10
Self Discipline

"Our greatest weakness lies in giving up. The most certain way to succeed is always to try just one more time."
— *Thomas A. Edison*

How Much Discipline Do You Have?

Self-discipline may be considered an art form and not one everyone has mastered. If you procrastinate or lack self-control in certain areas of your life, it's important that discipline is added to your life if you want to achieve happiness.

If you constantly do things against your better judgment and then live to regret it, you'll spend more time beating yourself up instead of being happy – and this is no way to live your life.

You may be your own person but you have to hold yourself accountable for what you do and what you feel. Without discipline, you are going down a path that is unrecognizable and one day, you will wake and wonder where you are and how you got there. Do not take this path. It is not a good one.

There are some important steps to teaching yourself discipline.

The first thing to be aware of is that you cannot constantly put yourself down for not being disciplined. Accept the fact that you need help and leave it alone. If you beat yourself up mentally over it, it's not going to help the situation.

Own up to it and move on. If you feel de-motivated, that's one thing. If you fall into a state of depression over your de-motivation, the problems have been made exponentially more difficult to overcome.

It's not unusual to become de-motivated. To err is human and this is something that you must remember at all times. It's going to happen. It takes time to learn new traits and master them, so don't focus too much on the failures. Focus on how to pick yourself up quickly and move on.

Why Discipline Yourself?

There is likely a goal that you need to achieve, and there will be obstacles in your way. Maybe you want to lose weight but really love food or want to get up earlier but have a habit of sleeping in late. It doesn't matter what it is. It can be overcome, but you have to decide what the "why" is behind it as this is going to become the ultimate form of motivation.

Once you have determined the "why", put it down on paper. Having the reminder can be important and keep you moving forward.

Now, create an action plan. Do it on a computer, on a dry erase board, or even in a journal. Focus on the form for the action plan before filling it all in. Include the goal and why at the top and then be sure you have room for:

- Action

- Timeline

- Obstacles

- Ways to overcome obstacles

- Progress

Take the time to start filling in all the sections on the form. This may take some time and that's okay because it's important that thought goes into each area. If you rush past the action plan, then the goal may never be met and now you have given yourself another reason to beat yourself up and fall into a state of depression. This scenario won't happen if you have an action plan that has been well thought out.

Start with Baby Steps

The action will be all of the steps needed to work towards the end goal; there may be as many steps as you want to get you to that level. Sometimes it can be easier to include more actions, as it will help you take the baby steps. Each one will feel like an accomplishment and provide the motivation to keep going.

The timeline is started when you want to start each action. Put some type of time limit on a goal. If you want to lose weight, what is the date you want to have to be 10 or 20 pounds lighter? If you want to save money, what is the date the money should be in your account?

There's always a time frame for doing things, so think about when you want to start and end. Fill it out in a calendar and have the reminders present so you don't lose track of what needs to be done.

Identify all the obstacles and be honest with yourself. What has stood in between you and your ability to achieve this goal in the past? Maybe you love to go out to eat or you work too long or the snooze button is calling your name. Whatever it is, get it down on the list.

Use Obstacles To Your Advantage

With a list of the obstacles, you can then work to make sure you figure out ways to overcome all these obstacles. If you struggle with waking in the morning because of the snooze button, consider moving the alarm clock so it's not right next to the bed.

There are always ways to overcome obstacles because they are simply obstacles. People go through obstacle courses all the time. It can also be beneficial to tell other people that you have goals and that you need help; ask them to help keep you on track. It helps to hold yourself accountable for meeting the goals; when you have to report to someone other than yourself, it can be the necessary motivating factor.

Track Your Progress

Progress is also something to keep up on. You have to look at where you are and how far you need to go in order to reach the goal. If you find yourself working backwards, don't panic. Identify it, identify the obstacle, and then work on those obstacles to continue moving forward once again.

Self-discipline comes from knowing what needs to be done and continuing forward. There will always be obstacles, but you cannot allow them to defeat you.

The plan that you have created needs to be implemented. It may take a few days to get into any kind of real routine. It may even take a few weeks. It can be a real struggle for a while, but once it has become second nature, following the plan will be easier than you originally thought. Don't let it get to you. Life will get easier when you can accomplish all your goals all the time.

Allow Others Experiences to Help You Succeed

Pull inspiration from others who had self-discipline. Milton Hershey, the founder of the Hershey chocolate company failed many, many times before making it big. If you have ever cherished biting into a piece of Hershey chocolate, you know all those struggles were worth the end result.

It's inspiring to see how many times he picked himself up and dusted himself off. He had faith in his ability to succeed and was surrounded by people pushing him forward, providing him with words of encouragement.

Milton Hershey isn't the only one with an underdog story of success. There are countless others and it can be advantageous for you to read some of them to see that it can be done – and these were all achieved because people learned the fine art of self-discipline.

Review Your Plan on Schedule

The plan that you created needs to be reviewed periodically. Make comments on the plan in terms of what is and isn't working. If there were areas missing in the original plan, go back and fill them out. If things didn't work, write in why and what can be done in the future.

Having some kind of written form can keep you on track and help you to make improvements the next time you have a goal to avoid the same obstacles over and over again. Learn from what you have done in the past and you may find it is easier to meet future goals because you have a plan.

Failure isn't a reason for depression. Failure can be a step to get you to your goal, especially if you have learned something from it. Life is full of lessons and you have to take an optimistic approach to meeting your goals because it will allow you to experience more happiness, even when the goals are not being met and even when obstacles have presented themselves.

Don't Give Up!

Whatever you do, don't give up. So what if you failed! Fine. Learn from your mistakes and keep going. If you beat yourself up too much, it's going to cause depression and the goal may never be met. It may be hard to stay motivated, especially when faced with obstacles, but it doesn't have to mean game over. Just pick yourself up and remind yourself that the goal is something really important.

Self-discipline is a great trait to have. The majority of people who have it started out without it. They worked on their discipline through action plans, through lots of failure, and then began seeing results. As you see more results on the way to your goal, all that is needed is the motivation and then your actions take over from there. It's best to focus on results than on any obstacles that may appear from time to time.

When you are able to practice a higher level of self-discipline, several things will happen. You will see more motivation and strength in yourself and find that it allows you to reach your goals. You will also be able to accomplish more and build the life you desire.

Think about what needs to be done for you to live the life you have always wanted. What would make you happy? Identify these and then begin building an action plan for each one. When you factor in the self-discipline factor, all these things are going to be feasible. As you accomplish each goal, you will find that you are happier and happier – and that happiness will grow as you get closer to having everything that you want in life.

Self-discipline can be applied to all aspects of your life. Your health, wealth, friends, career, and more can benefit from exercising self-discipline. As you surround yourself with a support group, they can help with the discipline and ensure you are moving forward without being too hard on yourself when obstacles appear from time to time.

Exercise 10. Setting Some Goals

1. Think about a goal you want to achieve in your life.

2. Write down why you absolutely want to achieve this goal.

3. Make an action plan for every week.

4. Every time you accomplish something, celebrate your milestone, and then move forward on your next action to do.

Chapter 11
Happiness at Work and Within Your Career

"The will to win, the desire to succeed, the urge to reach your full potential... these are the keys that will unlock the door to personal excellence."

— Confucius

Happiness needs to be found at the job that you have now, though this is not to say that you should be happy with status quo. Since you work, you should find happiness with the fact that you are employed. If it's not the job you want or even the job you need, happiness must still be found, with knowledge that it is a stepping-stone to something better.

Just because you are not in the career of your dreams doesn't mean you cannot be happy. Many people assume that as soon as they get into their ideal career that happiness will be instantly achieved. Often, this is the farthest from the truth.

Jobs Aren't Your Source of Happiness

Finding a good job will not instantly fix all the other reasons why you aren't happy. It's best to focus on how to get happy within your current job so as you do move up the corporate ladder and find the perfect job, you will know it and be able to experience the bliss that comes along with that.

A positive outlook allows you to make the best of any job, whether it is the best paying or even the one with the most meaning. If you have good relationships in and outside of the workplace, it will make it more enjoyable to go to work every day and then share your day with those who care most about you.

Whatever you do, do not use your job as a crutch. If you want to find meaning, then find meaning. But first, find happiness. Understand that your job can make you feel happy; finding happiness is entirely possible.

Is your job the best out there? No, probably not. Is your job inconsequential? No, absolutely not. You may not realize it, but your job has some level of meaning, even if it is not on the grand scheme you would like it to be. If you have a positive outlook about your job, it will allow you to have a more positive outlook on life.

How to Reframe Your Ideas About Work

Think about it. If you come home from work feeling miserable all the time, it impacts other things in your life. You may come home and be in a bad mood towards your family and your partner. This has a negative effect on your relationships. It means that instead of having a good relationship, you will have a bad one, even if things had been going well prior to you getting a job.

If you are negative and unhappy in one area of your life, it's only a matter of time before that negativity flows into another aspect of your life – and then another one and another one.

Your relationships are critical to your well being, and if you mess with those, you mess with the entire stability of your life and the ability to find happiness in all that you do.

Take a look at your job. Is it in the industry that you want to be in? If it is, take heart in the fact that you are at least in the industry where you want to be. Any job – in the medical field, sales, food & beverage, technology, or other field can be used as a stepping-stone to something bigger and better. The experience could prove to be invaluable – and you won't know it for years.

If you're not in the industry where you want to be, think about why you took the job that you're in. Maybe it's because you're going to school and the job fits into your schedule or because you are actively trying to break into a certain industry. Whatever it is, identify the reason why you are at the job you are at now and create an action plan as to how to get into the industry you want to be.

You are in control of your happiness. If you're not happy, then do something about it.

Your job/career should be making you happy because you spend so much time there. Without being happy with your job (and that means accepting why you're in it), then it's going to be impossible to be happy in other areas of your life. Come to peace with your job without losing that level of determination needed to seek the job you eventually want to have.

Maintain a positive outlook and focus on ways to improve your outlook at the current job – and watch how it can do great things for your life!

Your Soul Gives You Clues About Careers

Once you are on the right career path, you will feel it within your soul; it can be the fuel that's needed to be happy within the smaller jobs you must take along the way. Remember that nothing is going to happen instantly.

Sometimes you have to be patient and work your way up the ladder. You have to change a lot of bedpans before you become a nurse and you have to read a lot of books before you become a teacher.

No job is without its struggles but if you're on the right path, life will be better for you.

Exercise 11. Happiness in Your Career

1.   Are you happy with your career? If yes, write a paragraph on what you like in your working career, and feel grateful for that.

2.   If you are not happy or don't have a career yet, brainstorm on what you would like to do and what industry you want to be in.

3. Then write a plan on how you are going to achieve your dream career.

4. Read your vision every day and place it where you can see it. When you meditate, envision yourself having achieved your dream career. But remember, nothing happens overnight. You need to work every day toward your dreams and goals, and you need to do the work.

Chapter 12
Feelings of Happiness and Elation

"Always do your best. What you plant now, you will harvest later."
— *Og Mandino*

What is Happiness?

Happiness is defined as a mental state of positive and pleasant emotions. Many dictionaries define it as a state of well being. Note the term, "well" being used. You want to feel happiness as much as possible because it leads to a better form of being for you.

Elation is defined as extreme happiness, which is an even better emotion to have. If happiness leads to your well being, just imagine what elation is capable of doing! You can actually become someone who smiles constantly and always has something positive to say. It takes less effort than you might think.

Most people are already familiar with the law of attraction. It states that when you think positively, positive emotions and events will be sent your way. When you think negatively, negative emotions and events will be sent your way. It's better to get a promotion than be handed a pink slip. It's better to get an invitation to a wedding than a funeral and easier to spend time with happy people as opposed to sad or angry people.

Therefore, it is in your best interest to be happy. Happy people stay happy because they have the law of attraction working for them. You will be able to attract a lot of reasons to be happy when you have a positive way of thinking. The moment you stop thinking in a positive manner is when you are going to deal with an array of problems. You will then need to find your "happy place" in order to get back to where you were.

Can Life Get Any Worse?

Have you ever noticed that when things are bad, they are really bad? You may find yourself saying things like "Why this?" or "Can it get any worse?" This is because the law of attraction is working at full strength. The moment you let negativity in your life, that is all that you are going to attract and you may find it hard to attract anything else until you change your way of thinking.

Life is too short to focus on anything but being happy. You could wallow in your misery, but what is that really going to get you? Psychologists have claimed that being happy can add years to your life. This means that you can actually "will" your way into leading a longer and happier life just by focusing on a more positive perspective.

There are countless books out there about the law of attraction, which go into greater detail as to how you can use positive thinking to live the life you want to live. This includes learning how to turn bad situations into good ones and using positive comments as a way to fuel your way through the day. However you want to approach the topic is fine as long as you do so in a POSITIVE way.

Remember, feelings of happiness and elation impact your sense of well being, so it is in your best interest to experience them more often than not!

Understanding Emotions in Greater Detail

Walt Disney said, "If you can dream it, you can do it." Dreaming a goal is important but so are the emotions you have about your dream.

Emotions are more powerful than you might think and it's important to know how they are going to creep up when you least expect them. Life will always have surprises and a traumatic event can establish a considerable amount of negative emotions. When struck with something like this, you have to learn how to adapt.

There are also habitual feelings you have when you do very specific things. If you ALWAYS do a particular thing, there is a feeling associated with that. You have it each time it occurs and it may be difficult not to have this emotion. If it's a positive emotion, then it's a good thing, but what about the habitual feelings that you foster that aren't the good ones – like rage, doubt, insecurity, detachment, and others?

Understand the scale of human emotions. There are various emotions you can feel and they can be categorized in different ways. You can feel multiple emotions at the same time. Some of the categories include love, kindness, abundance, calm, wonder, courage, and worthiness.

If you don't feel love for something, the opposite is hate. However, there are other degrees within the category of love you may feel for someone as well, such as dislike, repulsion, or indifference. While you want to foster feelings of love or at least a like for everything and everyone in your life to be a happier person, you have to identify emotions effectively so you know what you are really dealing with.

It's important to be able to express emotions and then understand how you can overcome them. At work, how calm are you? Do you have a calm and quietness emotion or is it more like irritation, agitation, or even rage? If you have feelings of irritation or rage coursing through your body at work, it's not going to lead to happiness and excitement. Instead, it's going to result in more stress, more tensed muscles, and more misery.

How do you overcome emotions? You have to know where you are, where you want to be, and choose to make the change.

How Good are You At Overcoming Emotions?

Overcoming emotions is very difficult at times. If you have fostered hate for someone for so long, it's hard to let go and suddenly become very fond of the person. However, this doesn't mean that you can't move on.

Look at the details of the emotion and determine when hate first started. Do you really hate the person? Why? What did they do? Have you ever talked to this person about the hatred? What could be done to overcome the hatred?

I remember a time I was always angry about someone in my family, because I was expecting this person to be like me, driven, strong, determined, and money-conscious, but she was the complete opposite. I was mad about her and at her! Nevertheless this person was very genuine, loving, caring and honest.

The day I changed my expectation I had for this person, and began to appreciate her qualities, everything changed in a positive way! Instead of being mad about and at her, I was happy and grateful to have her in my life. Sometimes it's very easy and simple to change your emotions, you just have to switch your perspective of the world.

Know Why You Have Certain Feelings

These are all questions you have to ask yourself so you can get a deeper understanding of the emotion. Being able to identify your emotion on a scale of say 0 to 10 is only the first half. You have to know why you have these feelings so you know how to make some changes.

If you want to become a happier and healthier person, you have to let go of certain emotions because they are dragging you down. It is physically exhausting to loathe someone. You make an effort to avoid the person, not talk to him, and discuss him mentally in your head as to why you have the hate. You may even talk about him to others so that your displeasure is contagious.

Is this really worth it? Wouldn't your time be better spent ignoring the person altogether than to hate him in such a vigorous manner?

Slide Your Emotions Up the Ladder Towards Love

Think about how you can slide your emotions up the ladder towards love. If you hate him now, try to get to the level of indifference. At this point, you don't love him, but you don't hate him either.

Once you can get to this level, you can then make some efforts to find out things that you have in common so that you can like him. Over time, the relationship may evolve into love and that allows you to be happier when that person is in your personal space.

The same kinds of actions can be done about all the different emotions that you have. You want to be happy, calm, inspirational, confident, courageous, connected, and faithful. If you are not at these emotional markers, then you need to work towards them in all areas of your life.

Will it be hard? It depends on what levels of negative emotions you are at and how much time during the day you tend to be there. If you are happy until you go to work, you know you need to focus on improving your work environment. If you are courageous until it comes to talking to your boss, figure out what you can do to build up your courage.

Inner reflection can be an eye-opening experience to check in on what your emotional state is during the day. Identify the areas in your life where you need the most work and don't focus just on the emotion of happiness because there is so much more than that. You can be happy and still insensitive to someone's feelings.

Your Emotions Are Contagious

Remember that emotions are contagious. Are you doing all you can to embrace positive feelings? When you do this, more people are going to want to be around you. It is easier to be in a positive mood all the time because the people around you will also be in positive moods.

You can have a better life when you have positivity all around you. People will be smiling and offering words of encouragement instead of trying to be indifferent or even discourage you from your goals.

Think about how much more exciting it is to have cheerleaders in your corner for everything you do. In your life right now, you may have people who are dragging you down. If there are, think about yourself and whether you have been doing right by them. You may want to work on yourself before you judge anyone else. This one little tweak in consciousness leads to a life of fulfillment and joy.

Flipping the Switch on Your Emotions

Your emotions are there whether you realize them or not. Sense the emotions you have and then slow down for a few moments to contemplate what you are feeling at any given moment when you are by yourself (stressed, calm, etc.) as well as towards a certain person (love, indifference, hatred), and even towards particular goals or events (irritated, devoted).

When you understand your emotional state, you can make the switch on your emotions to improve them. Sometimes, though, you have to pretend as if you are flipping a switch.

Feelings of indifference are almost like saying that you have no emotion. You are indifferent as to whether a person lives or dies, you are indifferent to what is going on in your life, and you are indifferent in general. This is one of the worst emotional states to be in because you are not passionate about anything. There is no reason to live because you are indifferent to it all.

Part of what makes us human is our emotions and our ability to love and hate with equal vigor. While you don't want to turn the switch on to hate and tense emotions, it is a start in the right direction because it demonstrates your ability to feel something.

If you identify your emotions as indifferent, it could mean that you are suffering from a nervous breakdown. Those who are indifferent about multiple areas of their life are often severely depressed or suicidal. This is not a place you want to be because it's not a happy one. The good news is that you can get back into a situation where you are in control of your emotions and switch them back on by just making the conscious effort to live and to feel.

Do You Realize All the Control You Have?

You are in control of everything that goes on around you. You are in control of you. It's called free will. You choose how you want to feel and how you want to act. If you don't like your job, you make the choice to do something about it. If you don't like the people you hang around with, you make the choice to go out and find new friends. There is always a choice in your life, even if it is not obvious at the moment.

The choices you have to make may not always be the easiest. For example, if you are making only a small amount of money and you are not happy, making changes may seem harder because you don't have the money to just get up and transplant yourself to somewhere else. However, when you make the choice to be happier and flip on your emotions to care, you can start to do something about it all.

Emotions guide you through life. When you start to look at your life and where you want to be, that's a feeling of determination, which will drive you to where you want and need to be in order to be happy. You flip this switch to gain the drive. It's a better choice than choosing to be indifferent and not getting anywhere.

You choose to be happy. The choices are long-term and short-term, but you are the one making the choices in your life to work towards happiness. Knowing this can even make you happier because it means you have already accomplished a small portion of your goal. The only way to make any of this happen is to flip the switch on your emotions so you begin to feel and take control of the emotions that you are feeling.

Identify them. Work on them. Improve them until you reach a happy state of mind.

Evoke Emotions in Others

When you want to have more positive emotional experiences, think about those around you and what they would like. Giving gifts can be a great way to improve the happiness of those around you and improve yours as well.

The gifts don't have to be that extravagant. It can be something simple to tell someone you were thinking of them. You can even make the gifts if you wish as a way of being more personal (and saving money). If you have kids and your child has ever handmade a card or colored you a picture, it was from the heart and it made you smile. These things can do the same for those around you.

It's actually possible to feel more happiness for giving the gifts than the people receiving them will feel. You may not think much about it, but when you see someone else happy as a result of something you do, it can boost your dopamine levels, which is the neurotransmitter responsible for feeling happy. This means the more good you do, the more that neurotransmitter will be firing.

The gifts can be for people you know as well as for people you don't. Take a look at volunteering within your community. If you take note of how happy people are who are in charity work, the Peace Corps, and more, it is because they are doing something for other people. You can add a lot of joy in your life by helping others and it's because they are happy.

Whether you give the gift of an actual item or you give the gift of time, you are making it about someone other than yourself. As a result, they are going to be happy, which in turn makes you happy. When you get joy from helping others and giving to others, it's going to push you to do it with more frequency, keeping the positive cycle in motion.

As people notice the improvement in your mood and see you as happier, you can talk to them about what you're doing and get more people involved. When more people give to others, they will be happier as well – and it will all be as a result of what you have done.

The Pay It Forward Concept

Have you ever heard of the concept called "pay it forward"? It's the same principle. If you like someone doing something for you (giving you a gift, sending you a card, paying for your meal), then pay it forward to the next person – and hopefully it will continue so everyone is a giver instead of a taker. It can make the world a better place and keep a smile on your face.

You can also tutor and be a role model. You are being a help – and giving a child or an adult a clear path to their happiness as well. You cannot always think about yourself and when you choose to think of others, it leads to being compassionate. There are many children in the world who need tutoring, guidance, and general time with someone else. You can choose any number of organizations and charities where you can give your time and be a part of someone else's development – and they will be grateful to you.

Think about it. You have the chance to shape someone else's life. If someone isn't happy, you can take what you have learned and help them find happiness. When they find happiness, you find it as well. The two of you can bond over a mutual finding of a way to be happy in life – and it can form a bond that does not need to be replaced.

Find the Compassion in You

Compassion is an emotion to find within yourself if you plan on ever being truly happy. Create a vision for the world that avoids a lot of emotional reactions, but where you can see possibility. Don't feel sorry for people. Instead, do something about it.

If someone is hungry, feed him or her. If someone is thirsty, provide him or her with a drink. When you can provide nourishment in the form that people need, you become compassionate without feeling sorry or pity.

What's important is to ensure you are being compassionate for the purpose of wanting to help. Wanting to be a hero feeds some level of selfishness. You should want to help in order to be a good person. If you are doing good deeds for some ulterior motive, then it's not going to bring you true happiness.

You cannot look at the people you help and feel pity. Instead, you have to look at the people and know that what you are doing is making a difference and improving the person, the community, or the world in one way or another.

When you master compassion, it can be a humbling experience. You learn about another person or community or culture and see how they deal with the world. Accept life for what it is, but help where you can because you want to help and because you want other people to experience joy. It may not lead to happiness right away, but as you celebrate the small victories, it can be one of the best things you have every chosen to do.

A happy life is one filled with compassion that has nothing to do with selfish behaviors or expectations. Do because you love the feeling, not because you feel you have to or because you feel sorry for someone.

Exercise 12. Your Emotional Diary

1. In a journal, record and write down your daily emotions for one week.

2. For every negative emotion you experience, write a solution on how you can change it in a positive one. Be creative. And of course, if you feel lot of stress or frustration, start to exercise or meditate on a regular basis.

Chapter 13
Decide on What Works

"The secret of getting ahead is getting started."
— *Mark Twain*

You have been introduced to a variety of thought processes throughout this e-book. You have learned about the importance of positive thought, positive speech, eliminating toxins from your body, eating the right foods, meditating, practicing yoga, and unlocking physiology to release more endorphins.

All these could potentially help improve your level of happiness and help you achieve more positive emotions. Some techniques will be more effective for you than others, depending on who you are and what is going on in your life.

Search For Your Ideal Formula

There is no ideal formula, no matter what. Some people will be able to reach happiness without ever practicing yoga. Other people wouldn't dream of giving up their yoga for fear of being unhappy. You have to do what works for you. If you have yet to reach that point in your life where you know what makes you happy, you are going to need to test out a few different concepts that were covered.

It is all about doing what makes you happy. You have to focus on your own happiness before you can make anyone else happy. No one is telling you that you have to change your entire diet or quit your job because it doesn't make you happy.

You need to find a balance to foster a positive outlook on life. Sometimes, there aren't going to be any positives that are evident right away. This means that you have to meditate in one capacity or another to identify where the positive aspects lie.

It is not always going to be easy to identify what needs to be done. You can rely on others who already have a positive outlook and still use the tips and tricks within this book to assist you. You should always try a few new things periodically to see if they will give you the boost in energy or the positive outlook you have been reaching for.

While there isn't a set formula, you are now learning about what it takes to be happy at every level. You communicate in a positive way. You have a way to release stress from your body and your life in a way that is healthy. You fuel your body with the right foods so your body has more energy and operates more efficiently.

How Many of These Things Are You Doing?

You may be doing one or more of these things now, but are you doing all of them? You may be able to achieve some happiness because you communicate in a positive way. If you are not eating right, however, you are missing out on happiness from another level. The people who seem to be upbeat and happy about everything all the time are that way because they have achieved happiness on several levels. Maybe the way they were brought up is what gave them a good start or maybe that's the way they became after a lot of hard work.

Anything worth doing is worth doing right and that means take a close look at what you can do so that improvements can be made. Explore all the areas and be honest with yourself so you can begin making some needed changes within your life. Only then can you achieve the happiness you know that you want.

Exercise 13. What Makes You Happy?

1. Ask yourself what makes you happy each and every day.

2. Then practice it at least 3 to 4 times a week or daily.

Chapter 14
Positive Emotions Result in a Better Life

"Do you want to know who you are? Don't ask. Act!
Action will delineate and define you."
— Thomas Jefferson

It's been said before and it needs to be said again: Positive emotions result in a better life. When you are a happier individual, your life can be unbelievably exciting. However, if you have negative emotions, such as feelings of hatred or resentment, your life can be unbelievably miserable. When you look at the two side-by-side, is easy to see which one you would prefer.

Think about it in detail. There are a lot of positive emotions out there. The list includes:

- Happiness	- Glee	- Carefree
- Joy	- Devotion	- Adoration
- Grace	- Comfort	- Gratitude
- Certainty	- Unity	- Tranquility
- Peaceful	- Curious	- Enthusiastic

These are all feelings that are positive in nature. These are going to make you a happier and healthier person because you will have a better outlook on life. Anything and everything can be sweeter when you have these emotions thrumming through your body. It is easier to get excited about something, be thankful for something that happened, and even to bounce back from something that was less than ideal.

Pledge to Feel These Positive Emotions

All these feelings allow you to feel like you have a better life. Why not make the pledge to make your life better right now? The emotions you are feeling can be adjusted based upon how you think about things. You have already learned what you can eat and what you can say to yourself to make you feel better. You simply have to make the decision to do it.

If you are constantly feeling enthusiastic and curious, these feelings lead you towards bigger and better things. You won't be okay with status quo. You want to see what else is out there – and this could lead to many new adventures. When you are happy with the people you are with and you trust the people in your life, you can go on adventures and never have to worry about a disconnection or any kind of loneliness.

What to Do About Negative People

If you have ever been unhappy, you noticed that people do not want to be around you because it brings them down, too. Think about it in terms of what's going on in your life now. When you are happy and in a great mood, the last thing you want to do is be around someone who is negative. This is because they create a disconnection and dislike or even a repulsion wells up inside you. They may bring anxiety into your life, which leads to discontent and ultimately stress and unhappiness.

If you know people that are negative, you can choose to avoid them and eliminate them from your life. This is not always the easiest thing to do. What if your boss is one of them? While you may not be able to quit your job just because your boss is lonely and miserable, it does mean that you can work to adjust your own attitude.

You may begin to provide more sympathy and gratitude toward him or her to see if it improves their mood. If they have not made the decision that they want to be happy, they aren't going to get happy from an external source. This is something for you to identify so you can ultimately remove them from your life.

It may mean that you will start looking for another job. Look for another job? Is this going to make you happier? Is this going to lead to a better life? What if the boss there has worse problems with unhappiness?

If you are truly exhibiting positive emotions, the result is always a better life for you. This is because you are curious about what is out there. You have faith there is something better out there and you have confidence in yourself that you are capable of getting a better job.

The 6ᵗʰ Sense of Human Resources Managers

Human Resources managers are in their positions because they can sense confidence a mile away. When you go into an interview confident you are capable of doing the job and doing it better than anyone else, you are likely going to get the job.

When you are happy, and show that you are in a good mood, it can also demonstrate your abilities greater than anything that is on your resume, or anything you may say. This can also lead to higher pay scales, which means you traded a job where unhappiness was always lingering for something bigger and better.

Happiness is a True Choice

The truth is that happiness will always lead to a better life. You have to believe this in order for it to be true.

Every time you compare the positive feelings and emotions to the negative ones, you will pick the positive feelings. Why would you choose fear when you could feel excited? Why would you act indifferently when you could be involved in the decisions? Why be bored when there is always so much to do all around you?

This is an example of how to choose all the emotions you want to feel. While it is easy to say, "feel a different way." It can be as simple as making a choice.

Certainly, there will be occasions when you aren't in a positive mood from time to time. You may be tired and therefore feelings of indifference and even frustration will fill you. It is your ability to bounce back that will ultimately help you achieve happiness. This means that you need to be able to identify these feelings and know there is a way to reverse them.

For example, if you are starting to feel frustrated and indifferent, you can't feed into it. Instead, you have to make the mental note that you are feeling that way because you are tired. The solution to overcoming tiredness is to get some sleep. This may mean bowing out of a social engagement, just so you can get some much-needed rest – and it could be the best decision you make because when you return to your social engagements, you will be in a better mood – and more people will want to be around you because of your better mood.

Remember that moods are contagious. It is better to infect people with happiness and excitement rather than sadness and misery. The positive emotions you have will have positive effects throughout your life, so it's best to reach out for them to have the life you always wanted to live. Happier people are more successful – this means that it's the happiness that brings success, not success bringing happiness. If you want to be more successful in life, you have to start with obtaining more positive emotions in every aspect of your life.

The Law of Attraction and Its 11 Corollaries

Psychologists, religious leaders, and even New Age thinkers have talked about the Law of Attraction for years. It also got a lot of press in 2006 when a book called "The Secret" focused heavily on the idea.

The law is a simple one. You attract what you think about, regardless of whether it is good thoughts or bad thoughts. It is obvious you want to attract good things, which means you can control them with good thoughts. The moment you begin to think bad thoughts, you are likely going to attract bad things.

It's a way for the universe to establish a balance. There are good thoughts and events as well as bad thoughts and events floating all over the place. If you are in the habit of good and positive thinking, then good and positive events will take place in your life – and the opposite will happen if you are thinking bad and negative thoughts.

The truth can be seen quickly. Have you ever had a bad day where couldn't get out of your slump and then wondered, "Could this day get any worse?" What happened after that? If you're like most people, the day did get worse; the law of attraction was working full force. You had negative energy and negative events were attracted to you. Once you turned your thought process over to the positive, things started to look up for you.

There are various ways that the law of attraction will work for you or against you. Knowing these ways can ensure that you do what you can to think happy, positive thoughts to remain within the good graces of the universe.

Below are 11 different aspects about the Law of Attraction you may not realize.

1. You can focus on something enough to make it happen.

Everyone knows someone who is always talking about being sick – and that is the person who is always sick. This is because there is such a focus on it that it actually happens. The best thing to do is talk about being happy and that's what will come out of the situation.

The universe has a way of manifesting reality. If you continue to draw enough negative towards you, negative things are going to happen. They will be enough to give you a clue to change your paradigm and focus on positive, happy thoughts so that those are the things happening to you on a regular basis.

2. You can invite things into your life by thinking about them.

Your thoughts are alive and when you think about something you want, the desire grows stronger and stronger. This can be seen with people who want to run marathons as well as those who want to have an affair. If you think about it enough, it's probably going to happen. What this means to you is to make sure you keep your thoughts in check.

3. Thoughts are powerful and can become powerful.

You may have brought bad things into your life because you worried about them so much. This is because you are attracting events and creating your own reality. If you think about how much you want to accomplish something, it is probably going to get accomplished.

4. Learn to trust your instincts.

Everyone has intuition and it is within you so you can find it and will listen to it. Don't overthink things too much because it can lead to problems. Your emotions can show you the difference between right and wrong and that's a great way to attract happiness.

5. Good things can happen quickly.

One of the most powerful emotions is desire, and this is because of the focus and attention you give to them. When you want and desire something, it is possible to attract more positive actions about those things, which allows you to experience the things you want most in life.

6. You need to change perspective.

When you want to make a change, there must be visualization. You have to imagine how things should be and how you want them to turn out, not as they currently are. Whether you want to win an Olympic gold medal or get a promotion at work, you have to direct your thoughts into the desired direction.

7. Use dreams as a guide.

Your psyche may be trying to tell you something via a dream; it is up to you to listen. You can attract better things to you by listening to your dreams and taking action rather than ignoring them and worrying about what the dreams are about.

8. Improve your mental magnetism.

The law of attraction works by attracting things to you. Your magnetic power needs to be enhanced and this can be done with positive and powerful thinking. Whether you meditate, perform yoga, chant, or do something else, dedicate 10 to 15 minutes to thinking about your goals in life and the dreams that you want to see come to life.

9. Success is for everyone.

The law of attraction requires positive thinking to work to your advantage. If you want success, it's there for the taking. There is no law that says success is only for some people. There is an infinite supply of it, so attract some of it.

10. Don't dwell on the negative.

There are going to be disappointments and problems in life. You cannot dwell on the issues because it will only attract more things that will cause you more disappointment. Focus on the life you want and not the life that you have.

11. Don't watch shows that bring you down.

Negative energy can be picked up anywhere and you have to be cautious about how you let negative magnetism into your life. Many shows focus on crimes and disease. If you watch these negative experiences, you could be attracting them towards you without even knowing it.

Commit Right Now to Positive Emotions

The law of attraction works to your advantage when you have positive emotions. No one wants more misery and more discontent in their life, so be mindful about where you allow your thought to wander. If you obsess over various worries and problems, those worries and problems create a balance in their favor and send more things for you to worry and obsess over.

The moment your thoughts take a turn for the positive, you will begin to attract better things into your life. This means that you need to make sure magnetism is working in your favor instead of against you. It's simpler to do than you might think, so start making some changes in your life and remember that the law of attraction is always working, which means you always have to be on your game in regards to managing your emotions.

Place a reminder somewhere in your home or office to tell you to be more positive. Positive events, actions, and thoughts will create a positive vibe all around you. You will find that more positive things happen around you and this will lead to more happiness. The moment you think about or do something negative, follow it up with a positive thought or action so that the laws of attraction are working with you instead of against you.

Exercise 14. Appreciation is Great

1. Write an appreciation letter to yourself. Define yourself only with positive words and positive emotions.

Here's an example:

> Dear Adrian,
>
> I love you because you aren't afraid to take risks, try something new, and you have huge amounts of faith in yourself that you won't fail. And even if you did fail, you know that you'll make it through. I love you because you are such a loving, caring and altruistic human being, helping other people whenever possible.

Chapter 15
The Power of Purpose

"You don't have to be great to start,

but you have to start to be great."

— Zig Ziglar

There is power when you have purpose in life. Purpose is the reason you do or create something the reason for which something exists. Not having a purpose in your life could be what's preventing you from actually getting work done or reaching your goals. It can be advantageous for you to energize yourself and your goals using the power of purpose.

When you have a clear reason of WHY attached to every one of your goals, you have the motivation needed to move forward. This prevents the excuses and distractions that inevitably stand in your way. Think about why you are doing anything.

Why do you want to be happier? To be healthier and to be more social. The happiness question is likely an easy one to answer because everyone wants to be happier in one area of life or another. No one sets out with the intention of being miserable.

Step-by-Step Instructions on How To Create Purpose

Learning how to create the power of purpose in your life is easier than it might seem. You simply need to have some instructions on how to establish purpose...and remind yourself of it on a frequent basis.

Step 1: State your goal with a clear outcome.

When you state your goal, be as specific as possible. If you don't know the full outcome, this is something that you have to think about. How can you build any motivation to complete a task unless you know the desired outcome? The simple answer is that you cannot – and this is where many people fail.

A perfect example of this is college. People are told to go to college and off they go. Their goal is as simple as "go to college." They don't know the outcome because they haven't thought about it long enough.

This leads to people in undeclared majors, taking courses because it's expected of them. It then comes as no surprise when these same people don't graduate because they lack the motivation, or they graduate and go back to working the same job they always have because they didn't have a clear outcome for a major and a career.

This bad scenario can be avoided by learning to attach a clear outcome with every goal. The outcome and goal are mutually exclusive. Set up a rule for yourself: You cannot have a goal without an outcome or an outcome without a goal. This can be something that you formulate in your head or it can be something you write on a board that is visible to you through multiple times of the day.

Step 2: Define your purpose.

Why is reaching the goal so important to you? When you have reasons to support your actions, it will be easier to follow through. The example of going to college can be used. Why are you going? What is your purpose?

List as many reasons for wanting to go to college and graduate with a particular degree as possible. This will make it easier for you to have something to go back to when you need the motivation at various points in your life.

The more positive you are about the purpose, the easier it will be for it to come to fruition. Be specific and make sure that your definition makes sense for you. Remember to take other people out of the equation at this point.

Step 3: Be clear on the gain.

What do you have to gain by reaching this goal? Are you going to benefit socially? Monetarily? Think about how many ways you could gain from reaching the goal and list them all. You can also include ones that are based upon a series of events.

For example, if you do this, then ABC could happen and then DEF could happen. If you were to graduate college, you could by hired by a Fortune 500 company and you could later become the youngest CEO. Using "best case" scenarios can provide the added motivation that you need.

There are likely going to be various ways to gain by achieving your goal. You want to list all the gains so you have a list of reasons as to why achieving the goal is so important. As various things happen in your life, one gain may become more important than another – and having a list will ensure that the goal remains relevant so you do not need to go back to the drawing board.

Step 4: Be clear on what will happen if you do not achieve this result.

Some of the best motivation in the world comes from looking at what will happen if you do NOT reach your goal. You can choose to be as specific on this as you want to be. It can also help to be a little dramatic in terms of what could happen so you see what the worst-case scenario is. Life is full of surprises and there is no way of knowing what will happen if you don't reach your goal. By going to the extremes of the spectrum, you can give yourself a clear view as to what the worst thing could be.

What could happen if you don't finish college? You end up with large amounts of student loans and have no real-world skills to offer an employer. This leads to unemployment, student loan debt, and before you know it, you're living on the streets. This is a dramatic approach to not finishing college, but it has the potential to happen and may be enough to push you to reach your goal so no part of this becomes a reality.

Step 5: Think about the impact.

Your purpose may have the ability to impact other people in your life. You could impact one person or a long list of people. If you have purpose and are able to reach your goal, it could impact such people as:

- Family
- Friends
- Customers
- Community
- Political figures

By identifying the impact of your actions, you will be able to see the big picture. While you can only control yourself and what you do, your actions have the ability to impact others. Identifying the impact of your actions can provide additional motivation to make sure you take actions that are outside of your comfort zone so you provide a positive impact instead of a negative one.

All these steps can be combined to make sure that you establish purpose. You cannot hone in on the power of purpose without completing all the steps. Some steps will be easier to complete than others. If you want to harness this power effectively, make sure you think about it completely.

Write everything down and analyze the goal from every angle so you cover the topic deeply. Make sure you establish the most important reasons for completing a goal so you have the motivation needed to achieve the goal – and achieve happiness by adding a checkmark next to the goal.

Goal and Purpose

It's important to see how this works in real life. Listing out the steps works for some people, and for some people it is necessary to see how to apply these. You don't want to miss out on harnessing the power of purpose, which is why an example will demonstrate how goal and purpose are defined and established.

A common goal for people is to lose weight. To ensure the power of purpose is working with you, it needs to be anchored with a goal.

Goal: Lose weight.

Saying that you want to lose weight is a goal, but it is not enough. This is when you need to take it to the next level.

Be more specific about the outcome: Lose 20 pounds by December 31, 2015. This allows you to identify exactly when it must be done. Many people utilize SMART goals as a way of getting things done.

The Mnemonic SMART

SMART goals is a mnemonic. Each one of the letters stands for something different for you to identify so that you know that you have a quality goal in place.

S = Specific
M = Measurable
A = Action-oriented
R = Realistic
T = Time-based

When you have all these features, you know your goal is achievable and there's a deadline for accomplishing the goal. When there is relevance along with a deadline, you are likely to muster up more motivation to follow it through.

Next you need to identify the purpose. If you keep it as simple as "to lose weight", you are creating a circle that goes absolutely nowhere. Without a purpose, your goal is meaningless. By going through the SMART strategy, you can make your goal more specific and drive yourself forward with your goal to make it happen.

Why do you want to lose weight? Some common reasons for wanting to achieve this outcome include:

I must lose weight so my clothes will fit better.
I must lose weight so I can increase my energy and feel better.
I must lose weight so I will have more energy, need less sleep and have more time with my family.
I must lose weight and master health so I can climb a mountain with my children when we go on vacation.
I must reach a healthy weight and lifestyle to live long enough to enjoy my grandchildren and see them get married and established in their lives.
I must maintain a healthy weight and lifestyle to live long enough to play with my great grandchildren.
I must become a master of nutrition and energy to guarantee that my children grow up with health, exercise, nutrition and absolute 100% vitality ingrained into their psyche so they never have to deal with obesity, lethargy, addiction, disease, illness or prescription medication.

These will also become mantras you can use to give yourself positive self-talk to gain further motivation. The mantras, as discussed in a previous chapter, are great ways of psyching yourself up to take action when life is otherwise trying to bring you down.

Are You Your Own Cheerleader?

Sometimes the only person who will be your cheerleader is you, so be the loudest cheerleader around. Create the mantras that help you drive the outcome so you are more likely to follow through. If you cannot establish at least five reasons for reaching a certain goal, then you will likely be able to talk yourself out of obtaining the goal.

For example, if you allow too much negativity into your life, it's too easy to justify why you're not acting on a goal. How many times have you avoided losing weight because it was easy to say you couldn't afford new clothes? When you can justify one of the reasons for not taking action, you need to have other ones to fall back on.

If you can keep the list of reasons why you should accomplish your goal, there will be one reason you list that becomes the ultimate fuel for accomplishing your goal. Maybe it's that you want to be a better role model for your children or you want to improve your health so you live a longer, happier life. Whatever it is, you need to identify the REAL reason for wanting to achieve a particular goal.

In the morning, you need a reason to jump out of bed with the strength and motivation to carry out your goals. No matter what else is going on around you, you will have the drive to push forward and take action.

What happens when you reach your goal? You reach a higher level of happiness because you now have a sense of accomplishment. Many times, you become unhappy because you define yourself by your failures instead of your accomplishments.

You can turn this around easily enough by not allowing yourself to fail. You need to have the power of purpose driving everything you do so failure is not an option. When you have something powerful motivating you and pushing you to take meaningful actions, you will not allow yourself to fail.

It is important to remember that hitting obstacles and failing is not the same thing. You cannot control the obstacles that stand in your way. You can only control how you deal with those obstacles to ensure that they do not keep you from pushing forward for too long. When you have a reason and a purpose for completing a goal, it will be easier to push past the obstacles that come along so it doesn't even seem as though there is an obstacle.

How Would You React in This Situation?

Let's say that the gym near you closes down. This is an obstacle. It does not mean that you have suddenly failed in being able to lose the weight. When you have enough motivation, the gym closure is a stepping-stone to your goal.

You find another (better) gym or an exercise program that allows you to work out from home so you don't even need a gym to do your workouts. You determine how you reach your goal. If one door closes, there are plenty of others that will open – and if you have the energy and motivation to do so, you can continue down the path.

Let the Power of Purpose Work for You

Reaching goals leads to reaching happiness. When you have the power of purpose working for you, you can be a happier person even before you actually reach your goal because you know you are headed in that direction – and sometimes that is all it takes.

You have the ability to use the power of purpose in everything that you do. Regardless of whether you realize it or not, you have goals that need to be achieved. These can be as small or as large as you make them out to be.

Some goals are part of your personal life and others are involved in your business life. You may find that some goals cover both personal and business aspects – and the purpose of achieving the goals can be similar.

Empowering Questions To Ask Yourself Daily

On a daily basis ask yourself empowering questions like the ones below, to keep you focused on your purpose, and remind yourself on your WHY:

- Am I focused on my ultimate purpose every single moment?

- Do I really want to be happy in my life every single day?

- Am I standing guard at the door of my mind, in order to keep negative thoughts and belief out of my body?

- Am I practicing the Law of Attraction to take me closer to my ultimate purpose?

- If I get distracted or make a mistake, do I realign my focus and keep moving forward?

- Do I remember that doing mistakes are a regular process to be successful, as long as I learn from them?

- Will my ultimate purpose bring me joy, happiness and satisfaction?

- Am I having a healthy lifestyle, eating healthy food and exercising regularly?

These are Napoleon Hill's keys to success and fulfillment:

- Develop definiteness of purpose.

- Establish a mastermind alliance; be in proximity of successful people.

- Assemble an attractive personality.

- Use Faith in your purpose or vision.

- Go the extra mile; be willing to take massive action.

- Create personal initiative.

- Build a positive mental attitude.

- Control your enthusiasm by focusing on your dreams.

- Be self-disciplined.

- Think accurately.

- Control your attention.

- Inspire teamwork.

- Learn from adversity and defeat.

- Cultivate creative vision.

- Maintain health, making it a priority in your life.

- Budget your time and money.

"Sow an act, and you reap a habit. Sow a habit and you reap a character. Sow a character, and you reap a destiny." -Napoleon Hill

Chapter 16
Bringing it All Together

"I know where I'm going and I know the truth, and I don't have to be what you want me to be. I'm free to be what I want."

— *Muhammad Ali*

We covered a lot throughout this book and it's important to work on everything instead of picking and choosing. Achieving balance within your life is important if you want to be happy and maintain happiness. This means you have to consider how to make improvements within all aspects.

If you only work on you instead of your relationships and your career at the same time, the happiness is going to be short-lived because you won't have the support that is required – and people who drag you down will appear again. Happiness is something that can occur throughout your life and if you go chapter by chapter, there are lessons to be learned and tips to follow.

When you believe in yourself, show compassion to others, learn to speak positively to yourself and those around you and figure out how to relieve stress, happiness is going to be within your reach. Once you have the happiness, it is up to you to hold onto it for as long as possible. When you have focused on all areas of your life, holding onto the happiness is easy. You can become the person people look up to, inspire to be, and ultimately want to be around.

Map Our Goals to Prevent Failure

Mapping out your goals and defining purpose for each goal may seem time-consuming, but it is a sure way to achieve happiness. The whole purpose of this book is to make sure that you know how to become happy. If you are unable to reach goals on a regular basis because you find one reason or another not to make them happen, you are never going to reach the full level of happiness that you want to reach.

Failure happens too often because there is no reason for reaching a goal. You don't want to be one of those people that reach an obstacle and suddenly stop because you don't have the motivation to push past the obstacle. No matter what, there are going to be obstacles throughout your life. How you choose to overcome them is up to you. All you need is a little extra motivation to help push past them in an effortless manner so you can start to reach more goals.

If you don't think it is possible, try it out. When you have purpose, you have motivation. When you have motivation, there is nothing stopping you from reaching any of your goals, no matter how small or large, they may be. This is because you have the motivation to figure out how to go around the obstacles and limit the obstacles that stand in your way.

Don't Be Afraid to Rely on Others

Expect to have instances when you need to rely on others to help you achieve your goals. This can be a personal trainer, a mentor, a political official, or someone else. When you have demonstrated the power of purpose, people will be able to sense it about you. When you have the power of purpose driving your goals, there are going to be more people willing to join you on your journey because they know that you are not going to fail, no matter what.

If you stand behind your beliefs and focus on the end goal, many people will want to help you, push you, and be there to see the results along with you. By bringing in additional people, you can also make sure that you are accountable to those individuals – and the desire inside of you to not fail in front of others may be another driving force to help you reach your goal.

Lists Will Help You

Whether you list out your goals and purpose for reaching goals on paper, type them out on the computer, or place them up on some kind of motivational board, it is important to spend the time listing them out. This will ensure no excuses crop up for not completing a goal. Your happiness is in your hands. There are steps that you can take to make sure that you achieve happiness, no matter what.

Go ahead and write down what needs to improve. If you write it down, you can see what you need to work on and that will make it easier to figure out how to achieve happiness. There may be some areas that need more work than others. Happiness may not happen immediately, but you can start taking measures that will allow more joy into your life slowly until you begin experience happiness on a daily basis. You can become an optimist and the type of person people pull strength from because you can find the joy in everything.

Chapter 17
Maintaining the Happiness

"If you don't design your own life plan, chances are you'll fall into someone else's plan. And guess what they have planned for you? Not much..."
— *Jim Rohn*

Throughout this book, you learned about happiness and why it is so important in your life. The only way to maintain the happiness is to focus on it every day. You have to make the decision to be happy. When you put your mind into your emotions, you can choose to be a happier person.

This is done through the way that you speak to yourself, to others, and even what you feed to your body as fuel. At the end of the day, you are the only one responsible for whether you are happy or not. You cannot look to others to make you happy. When you start to look to others, you may only find misery.

Not everyone is happy and not everyone will get happy because it is a decision they have made themselves and have chosen to live with. This does not have to be you. You can be happy. You know what you have to eat, what you have to say, and how to look at life in a positive way. The only thing left to do is maintain that happy feeling so that you can have a brighter, more enjoyable life.

Don't Worry – Be Happy!

Bobby McFerrin had it right when he sang the words "Don't worry; be happy." He promoted happiness to the world as he sang the lyrics over and over again – and many people took his advice. They stopped worrying and they started to focus on ways to experience happiness. Throughout this book, you learned about various ways you can be happy AND healthy.

When you're not happy, you're going to become stressed. Being stressed leads to such things as ulcers, problems with digestion, and countless other degenerative diseases. This means that when you are not happy, you are not healthy. What can you do about it? Get happy!

Maintaining Happiness: 9 Tricks to the Trade

You should know how to get happy by now, but how do you maintain it? There are some tips and tricks that happy people use so they can continue to be happy regardless of what is happening around them. If you want to be happy and stay happy, learn these tips and tricks for yourself to experience this feeling of well being for your entire life.

1. Remember to say "thank you" often (and mean it).

   This may seem very simple, but people of all ages forget to say it. These are two of the simplest words to utter and it helps you to express gratitude towards others. When someone says or does something that helps you or compliments you, be sure to say those words. It can not only promote happiness but also shift you away from bitterness and despair.

   If you don't have someone to say "thank you" to, then come up with a reason to be thankful for the day. Say it out loud and write it on a dry erase board or somewhere that you can see it through the whole day.

2. Forgive people.

   Holding grudges is not a healthy thing to do. Life is too short to have a bitter attitude towards someone or even to resent him or her for what he or she do or what they have done. It can affect you physically as well as mentally, so learn to be more altruistic and forgive people.

If you are having a particularly difficult time doing this, hold a conversation with them. Recall the hurt and explain why you are feeling this way. The person that you need to forgive may not realize that they have hurt you and send an apology your way, making it easier to move past the event.

Tell the person you forgive them and hold onto the forgiving feeling as opposed to holding onto the hurt and anger. If you choose not to forgive, it can lead to chronic stress and this can lead to anxiety and depression.

3. Turn negative into positive.

Negative things will happen in your life. There is no way of getting around these. However, you cannot dwell on the negative. When you learn to put a positive spin on the events that are negative, you can find happiness faster and this is going to lead to a better level of mental health all around. You are only going to feel helpless and inadequate if you let the negative events drag you down, so figure out how to make it positive.

If you have been laid off from work, look at it as an opportunity to find a better and higher paying job. If you have learned you are sick, look at it as an opportunity to improve upon your health and get the rest and relaxation you have needed. There is always a silver lining or a light at the end of the tunnel with every situation. Happy people find these things quickly so that they can be more optimistic.

4. More money doesn't mean more happiness.

Those with little money think that more money will get them happiness. Hopefully by now, you know that is not the case. If you keep poisoning your body, you aren't going to be happy no matter what because you won't be as healthy as you can be. Whether you are below the poverty line or making six digits a year, you can feed your body good food – and that can lead to happiness.

The same goes for positive thinking. There is no money in the world that will buy you the ability to suddenly be able to think positively. This is something you have to make the decision to do. People who are poor can think positively and people who are millionaires can think negatively. Money doesn't impact this.

The sooner you realize that money isn't going to help you, you will be happier (and healthier) for it. That doesn't mean that it can't help you relieve stress, however. This is the caveat. Money won't buy you happiness, but it can help you reduce some of your stress. A few examples are treating yourself to a massage once a month or going on a vacation where you can forget about the worries of the world for a week or so.

There is a way for you to get these things even without having a lot of disposable income. The solution is to save. Create a savings account or even a piggy bank and put a few dollars in each week. If you cut out eating out or coffees at the coffee shop in the morning, you can contribute even more. That money, accumulated over time, can be a great way to sneak in some fun and relax. Knowing that it's there should be enough to make you a little happier knowing that you have future fun in the process.

5. Create a calming environment.

Have you ever walked into someone's home and felt instantly at ease? This is because they have established a calming environment. You can call it feng shui or anything else, but it is a way of ensuring that you are comfortable. Large open spaces without a lot of clutter can help you breathe deeper.

If you can block out some of the noise of your surroundings with a bubbling fountain or some soft music playing, it can also help to calm your nerves. You don't want to feel as though you are in an elevator, but a day spa would be a good goal to shoot for. Organizing your desk can do wonders for your stress, which in turn does wonders for your ability to become happy. Get rid of the piles of work around you, even if it means filing them and reaching in for small stacks at a time.

The environment you are in will have a direct impact on your over-all happiness; so don't let something that you can change be the very thing that brings you down. A few minutes of adjusting things can go a long way to making sure you have what you need to bring a smile to your face.

6. Boost your energy levels.

You already know that certain foods affect your moods. You may need a boost of energy in order to feel happier. If you don't have energy, it's hard to let pessimism in because you are dragging your-self around. You may want to go for a walk, stand up and do some stretches, or eat some food that is good for your body. Nothing has to stand in your way of doing this.

If you sit at an office all day, take the time to get up from your desk and go for a walk, even if it is something as simple as taking three or four trips to the copy room. Research has shown that metabo-lism is faster in those who move faster. It's going to be better for your mood, so just work on improving your energy levels just a notch and see what happens.

7. Spend time in the sun.

Getting a tan doesn't necessarily result in happiness, but the sun does have an effect on your personality. Think about days where you have been in the sun versus days when you have been locked in an office with no access to daylight. What days are you the hap-piest?

The sun can affect your mood and if you don't have an office with a window or the blinds or shut, this may be part of the problem. You don't want to be grumpy just because you're not in the sunlight, so make a few changes so that you are. Maybe the remedy is having lunch at an outdoor café on your break or maybe it is taking a stroll at the top of every hour out to your car so that you can absorb some of the rays and put a smile on your face at the same time.

8. The key to maintaining happiness is becoming more optimistic.

You don't have to be the most optimistic person out there, but it pays to be more optimistic as opposed to being pessimistic or even realistic. Many people who say they aren't pessimistic are simply being optimistically pessimistic. If the glass is only filled half of the way, it's better that there is something in there than nothing at all, so you might as well look at it as half full.

It goes back to being grateful for the things you have and that means you should be grateful that your glass is at least half full. If you spend all of your energy hoping that your glass was full to the rim like other people you know, the thoughts lead to negative thoughts, depression, and eventually take a negative toll on your health.

9. Combine what you have learned.

Becoming happy involves combining various aspects of what you have learned throughout this book. While you should always be eating healthy, it is also important to engage in meditation, yoga, and think before you speak to others. There is no formula that is perfect for everyone. You have different things going in your life than others do and you need to learn how to manage them effectively.

If you are already eating in a healthy manner and are not achieving happiness, then consider various other tactics to implement. Maybe the solution is spending some time meditating each evening or surrounding yourself with happier people so you are not brought down by the problems and worries of others. Regardless of what you do on a daily basis, take action to achieve happiness because it is not going to find you on its own.

How long the happiness is maintained is completely up to you. This eBook is designed to help you become happier and healthier, but it won't prevent you from dealing with negativity or pain in your life. Bad things will happen but how you bounce back from them will be a testament to your attitude. You control your happiness and nothing else and no one else can take that away from you.

When you are happier, you have a better time throughout life. You are healthier because you don't have stress taking its toll on your body and you will generally have better relationships. Remember that happiness attracts happiness because the law of attraction says so. This means that it's in your best interest to be happy.

Various tips were provided throughout this eBook and they can help you to achieve happiness more often by showing you how to put in the extra effort within various aspects of your life. A happier you is always a healthier you, so go ahead and give it a try. Don't think that you can't do it because you can – and you will be much better off when you take the plunge and decide that happiness is a feeling that you would like to experience.

Good luck and start being happy!

"Never, Never, Never give up." – Winston Churchill